Journal (

Anthrozoos

A multidisciplinary journal of the interactions of people and animals

Produced in cooperation with the Humane Society of the United States (HSUS),
American Humane Association, American Society for the Prevention of Cruelty to Animals,
WALTHAM, and the International Association of Human–Animal Interaction Organizations (IAHAIO)

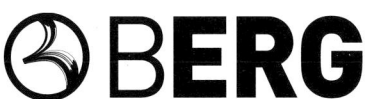

Anthrozoös (ISSN 0892-7936 print; ISSN 1753-0377 online) is published four times per year by Berg Publishers, 50 Bedford Square, London WC1B 3DP, UK. Four issues form a volume.

2012 Subscription Rates
Print and Online
Institutional: £254/ $494 (1 year);
                 £357/ $695 (2 year)

Online Only
Institutionall: £216/ $419 (1 year);
                 £304/ $589 (2 year)

Free online subscription for institutional print subscribers.

Full color images are available online.

Access your electronic subscription through www.ingentaconnect.com

2012 Membership Rates
Individual = £69/ $125

Society Affiliates = £69/ $125

Student Affiliates = £33/ $60

Corporate Membership = £207/ $375

Lifetime Membership = £1,375/$2,500

Members and Affiliates of the International Society for Anthrozoology (ISAZ) receive the journal as part of their membership package.

Individual membership of the ISAZ is open to individuals currently or previously involved in conducting scholarly research within the broad field of human–animal interaction. Individuals who have an interest in the field of human–animal interactions, but who have not conducted scholarly research in the field, may apply to become Society Affiliates. For further details and to apply for membership, please see www.isaz.net.

Institutional Orders and Payment
Turpin Distribution handle the distribution of this journal. Institutional orders accompanied with payment (checks made payable to Turpin Distribution) should be sent directly to Turpin Distribution, Stratton Business Park, Pegasus Drive, Biggleswade, Bedfordshire SG18 8TQ, UK
Tel: +44 (0)1767 604951
Fax: +44 (0)1767 601640
E-mail: custserv@turpin-distribution.com

Indexing
Articles appearing in this journal are abstracted and indexed by Abstracts in Anthropology; Animal Behaviour Abstracts; CAB Abstracts; Cumulative Index to Nursing and Allied Health Literature; Current Advances in Ecological and Environmental Sciences; Current Contents/Social and Behavioural Sciences; EMBiology; Environmental Periodicals Bibliography; Focus on Veterinary Science and Medicine; Geobase; Indian Journal of Veterinary Medicine; Linguistics and Language Behaviour Abstracts; Psychological Abstracts; Referantivnyi Zhurnal: Biologiia; Science Citation Index Expanded; Scopus; Social Science Citation Index; Sociological Abstracts; Veterinary Bulletin.

Berg Publishers is a member of CrossRef

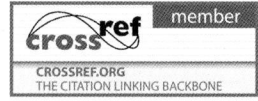

Information for advertisers
Advertising orders and inquiries may be sent to:
Berg Publishers, 50 Bedford Square, London WC1B 3DP, UK.
Tel: +44 (0) 207 631 5600
Fax: +44 (0) 207 631 5800
E-mail: Eleanor.Graves@bloomsbury.com

Prepress production by Communicating Words & Images, Seattle, WA, USA.
E-mail: andrealeighptak@me.com

Printed in the UK

Journal of the International Society for Anthrozoology

anthrozoös

A multidisciplinary journal of the interactions of people and animals

Volume 25, Issue 1, March 2012

CONTENTS

ANTHROZOÖS VOLUME 25, ISSUE 1 REPRINTS AVAILABLE PHOTOCOPYING © ISAZ 2012
P. 4 DIRECTLY FROM PERMITTED PRINTED IN THE UK
THE PUBLISHERS BY LICENSE ONLY

EDITOR'S THANKS

During 2011, many people helped me by either refereeing articles, writing book reviews, or providing information for "News & Analysis." Thanks to all these people:

Cindy Adams	Anne Eckhardt	Brinda Jegatheesan	Harriet Ritvo
Teri Allendorf	Marie-José Enders-	Rebecca Johnson	Melanie Rock
Patricia Anderson	Slegers	Edo Knegtering	Diane Rodgers
Sandra Barker	Amy Fitzgerald	Sarah Knight	Bernard Rollin
Mara Baun	Clifton Flynn	Lori Kogan	Mo Salman
Alan Beck	Jay Foreman	Cynthia Kosso	Catherine Schuppli
Lisa Beck	Lisa Freund	Kurt Kotrschal	James Serpell
Andrea Beetz	Alan Fridlund	Mai Kuha	Jo-Ann Shelton
Pauleen Bennett	Erika Friedmann	Gina-Anne Levow	Tania Signal
Penny Bernstein	Robert Garner	Julie Levy	Valerie Sims
John Bradshaw	Nancy Gee	Randy Malamud	Margaret Slater
Marc Brightman	Andrew Gilbey	Vanessa Malcarne	Birgit Stetina
Eric Brown	Benson Ginsburg	Linda Marston	Arran Stibbe
Sue-Ellen Brown	Theresa Goedeke	Garry Marvin	Trevor Stokes
Clare Browne	Sam Gosling	Andrew McLean	Rosemary Strasser
Brenda Bryant	Jessica Greenebaum	Vicky Melfi	Jo Swabe
Gordon Burghardt	Aaron Gross	David Mellor	Jill Taggart
Jonathan Burt	Eleonora Gullone	Gail Melson	Nicola Taylor
Rebecca Cassidy	Lynette Hart	Ádám Miklósi	Adrienne Thomas
Alexandra Chambers	Mark Haywood	Robert Mitchell	Clem Tisdell
Elizabeth Cherry	Susan Hazel	Claire Molloy	Ann Toohey
Matthew Chin	Paul Hemsworth	Paul Morris	Susanne Waiblinger
Nicholas Christenfeld	Bill Henry	Erin Myers	Paul Waldau
Juliet Clutton-Brock	Andreas Hergovich	Jenny Newman	Debbie Wells
Grahame Coleman	Hal Herzog	Mark Orams	Joan Wharf Higgins
Marion Copeland	Gail Holst-Warhaft	Elizabeth Peel	David Williams
Anna Chur-Hansen	Zsuzsanna Horvath	Rose Perrine	David Wilson
Beth Daly	Yuying Hsu	Anke Prothmann	Wendy Woodward
Margo DeMello	Carroll Hughes	Michael Ramirez	James Yeates
Diane Dutton	Melissa Hunt	Hayley Randle	R. Lee Zasloff
	Leslie Irvine	Ryan Rhodes	

Special thanks to Andrea Ptak, who deals with copy layout and proofs, and to Ken Bruce, who oversees the production of the journal at Berg Publishers, for their excellent work.

Finally, all at *Anthrozoös* deeply appreciate the generous financial support provided by WALTHAM, Humane Society of the United States, the American Society for the Prevention of Cruelty to Animals, and the International Association of Human–Animal Interaction Organizations.

ANTHROZOÖS   VOLUME 25, ISSUE 1   REPRINTS AVAILABLE   PHOTOCOPYING   © ISAZ 2012
              PP. 5–23   DIRECTLY FROM   PERMITTED   PRINTED IN THE UK
                             THE PUBLISHERS   BY LICENSE ONLY

Bystander Apathy in Animal Abuse Cases: Exploring Barriers to Child and Adolescent Intervention

Arnold Arluke
Department of Sociology, Northeastern University, USA

Address for correspondence:
Professor Arnold Arluke,
Department of Sociology,
Northeastern University,
Boston, MA 02115, USA.
E-mail: aarluke@gmail.com

ABSTRACT The present study examines how children and adolescents respond when witnessing animal abuse and why many do not intervene to help animal victims. Ethnographic interviews were conducted with 25 late adolescents who witnessed animal abuse months or years earlier. Results were generally consistent with, but not identical to, findings from previous research on bystander intervention with human victims. On the one hand, the response of bystanders to animal abuse was similar to that of bystanders witnessing violence against humans. Both kinds of bystanders are very troubled by what they witness but often appear to be indifferent to the distress of victims, saying or doing little if anything to stop victims from being harmed or to prevent perpetrators from repeating their violence. On the other hand, while both types of bystanders faced the same general barriers to helping, the nature and salience of these barriers differed when comparing the two groups. Child and adolescent bystanders of animal abuse, unlike bystanders of human violence, were heavily deterred by a definition of animal abuse as a form of play among peers that normalized violence and included bystanders as participants, the fear of being labeled a tattletale or spoilsport if bystanders reported the abuse to others or caused it to stop, and individual attitudes and beliefs that led bystanders to excuse or justify the abuse or to feel as though they had no support for protesting, reporting, or preventing it. Implications of the findings are discussed for educating children and adolescents to intervene on behalf of abused animals.

Keywords: animal abuse, bystander apathy, child and adolescent helping behavior

 Despite long-standing interest in promoting humane behavior, researchers have failed to examine real-life situations where children and adolescents could, but often do not, behave altruistically to help animals that are intentionally harmed, neglected, or otherwise left in distress by peers, family members, or strangers. Like their counterparts

Anthrozoös   DOI: 10.2752/175303712X13240472427753

who witness human victimization, it is disturbing to hear about children and adolescents who witness the victimization of animals but do nothing to stop their harm, provide them care, or prevent subsequent acts by perpetrators. Yet with human victims, researchers have spent decades trying to understand the roots of such youthful bystander apathy, while completely neglecting this question when the victims are animals. What barriers prevent children and adolescents from helping animals in distress and to what extent, if at all, is their behavior any different from the response of bystanders to human victims?

Rather than asking these questions, researchers have focused on the long-term impact of witnessing animal abuse. Some have studied the trauma of seeing cruelty and its affects on the witness's emotional and behavioral development, suggesting that observing animal cruelty might lead to problems such as increased rates of missing school or decreased empathy (e.g., Kolbo, Blakely and Engleman 1996). Others have examined the connection between observing animal cruelty and how this might affect future caring or cruelty to animals, reporting confusing results, as noted by Daly and Morton (2003).

Research on bystander apathy with human victims can guide the analysis of, and provide a comparison for, this behavior in animal abuse cases. Three general barriers to helping have been identified by researchers. One type of barrier is situational; rather than being indifferent to the victim's plight, bystanders respond to other observers and the group context within which the emergency or violence occurs (Latane and Darley 1968). For example, social norms, especially those emerging during the event, can be a major source of bystander apathy because others present may expect bystanders to not intervene. Bystanders also can feel pressure to view the unfolding event in ways that normalize violence and suffering.

Cost-reward barriers stem from bystanders balancing how much they think the victim needs help against the costs of helping (Piliavin et al. 1981). If bystanders believe that the personal cost of helping (e.g., how much time and effort it will take) is much higher than the cost of not helping, then they will usually not intervene. If the personal cost to bystanders is low, then bystanders will usually intervene (Clark and Word 1972; Howard and Crano 1974; Shotland and Stebbins 1983; Bell et al. 1995).

Finally, individual barriers stem from bystanders' background, personality, and character. On the one hand, personal norms or feelings of moral obligation to behave in a particular way in specific situations have been found to influence helping behavior (Schwartz 1977) and a person's sense of strength, efficacy, and competence to deal with violence and aggressiveness also appears to make intervention more likely (Huston et al. 1981; Rigby and Johnson 2006). However, other research shows no relationship between the likelihood of intervening and certain character traits, including being empathic, sympathetic, nice, and caring (Rabow et al. 1990).

It is unclear whether or how these three barriers apply to children and adolescents witnessing violence against animals, since existing research on bystander behavior examines human victims and typically focuses on adult bystanders in laboratory rather than real-life situations. Intervention may be even more difficult for younger bystanders because they are more influenced by social pressure to conform (Costanzo and Shaw 1966) and to win peer approval and membership (Espelage, Holt and Henkel 2003; Bauman 2007) than are adults. And intervention may be less likely with animal victims because they cannot ask for help, do not exhibit distress in ways easily understood by onlookers, are usually accorded less social worth than humans, and are not known by many people to be protected by anti-cruelty statutes enforced by humane law enforcement agencies.

Exploratory qualitative research can begin to assess the applicability of these barriers to child and adolescent bystanders of animal abuse. Results would not only redirect the attention of scholars to this promising new research direction but also offer vital information to anti-violence programs aimed at making junior and high school students more sensitive and responsive to animal cruelty. If these programs knew the barriers that prevent child and adolescent bystanders from helping animal victims, they could teach participants how to circumvent these barriers and potentially interrupt animal abuse in progress or even prevent future victimization. For example, information about these barriers could improve the accuracy and realism of teaching tools used in these programs, such as the use of hypothetical animal cruelty scenarios. In addition, if we knew why some children and adolescents choose to intervene in these situations, these programs could better pinpoint exactly what attitudes and beliefs might be instilled or amplified in participants to more effectively empower them to intervene.

Methods

A convenience sample of 25 adolescent bystanders of animal cruelty was drawn from eight introductory anthropology and sociology classes at a large urban eastern university in the US, representing five percent of the total enrollment in these classes. The author read a prepared statement to each class soliciting volunteers to participate in this study if they had witnessed but not caused physical suffering or death to animals, excluding hunting, animal experimentation, and pest/nuisance control.

Demographically, the mean age of the respondents was 19 at the time of the interview. Respondents' ages when they witnessed cruelty ranged from eight to 18 years old; given their ages at the time of the interview, a few interviewees were recalling incidents that took place as long as a decade earlier or as recently as a year, but for most, the witnessed incidents were approximately three to five years prior to the interviews.

About half the respondents were female and all but one was white. The vast majority were liberal arts and science majors, while others majored in business, engineering, or physical science.

In terms of bystander behavior, about half the respondents were non-interveners who failed to say or otherwise act to stop the abuse during or after the observed cruelty. Interveners represented the remaining half of the sample, either saying or doing something to stop the abuse. The majority of respondents witnessed cruelty to rodents (65%), while a minority saw it inflicted on dogs and cats (20%), reptiles (10%), or birds (5%).

Respondents were interviewed in private for approximately 45 minutes to an hour after obtaining informed consent. The unstructured and open-ended taped interviews asked respondents to describe the cruelty incidents, to recall their feelings, thoughts, and actions during the incidents, and to reflect on why they said or did certain things, or failed to do so, at the time or subsequent to it. After transcription, a grounded theory approach was used to identify themes in the data set.

One possible study limitation is the sample. Results may be culturally limited, given that almost the entire sample was white and upper-middle class. Although there is no corresponding data on animal abuse and bystander behavior among inner-city youth, research on race, ethnicity, and class differences in response to violence toward humans suggests that such demographic differences might also influence the present study (Towns 1996; Warner and Weist 1996; O'Campo, Shelley and Jaycox 2007). An additional concern about the sample is that it might overrepresent the proportion of interveners in the general population. Some animal non-interveners may tacitly or even explicitly approve and support the perpetrators' acts at the time of the event. If so, these non-interveners might be reluctant to participate in this study for social desirability reasons, if they think the author would criticize their encouragement of cruelty. Correspondingly, interveners might be more willing to participate because of the social desirability of helping behavior.

Another possible limitation is that some students had to recall events from years earlier. Retrospective accounts can be faulted for their inaccuracy, since details of the events can be forgotten or distorted over time. However studies on the accuracy of recalling traumatic events report that bystanders have very accurate memories of untoward and violent situations (Christianson, Goodman and Loftus 1992; Heuer and Reisberg 1992). In addition, the gap in time had its advantages because it gave interviewees enough distance to comfortably talk about former events and to critically reflect on what had happened.

Finally, rather than gathering accurate data on the sources of bystander apathy, asking interviewees about why they did not intervene might have only elicited excuses or justifications because they were asked to reflect on their prior decision-making in front of the author and from the perspective of young adults who were now uncomfortable with, or even ashamed by, their prior behavior. However, given the limits of retrospective interviewing, it is impossible to distinguish whether interviewees' comments were mere excuses and justifications or reasonably accurate descriptions of their prior thinking, feeling, and behavior.

Results

Virtually all interveners and many non-interveners shared something in common: a feeling of emotional and/or moral distress, sometimes substantial, when observing animal abuse, a desire to see it stop, and a hope to not see it repeated. Having this humane response, however, did not always translate into intervention and, when it did translate into intervention, it did not always translate into clear-cut helping behavior that stopped the abuse or thwarted its repetition. To understand this gap between humane response and action, I will first describe the kinds of interventions taken by some interviewees and then discuss what barriers tempered or prevented their interventions.

The Interventions

Despite being disturbed or saddened by the abuse they witnessed, most interviewees said or did nothing to stop it or prevent the abusers from doing it again. Forty percent of the interviewees (10) remained on the scene during the abuse, watching in silence, giggling out of nervousness, or making comments like "wow" that were perhaps wrongly interpreted as support by others present.

Thirty-two percent of the interviewees (8) said something to the abusers that might have been intended to express criticism but was not delivered in an effective and clear manner. Many of these interviewees spoke in hesitant ways, reminiscent of the hesitant resistance of the subjects in Stanley Milgram's (1974) classic experiment on obedience. These interviewees only said something once or twice to the abuser and worded their criticism in oblique ways, using humor or posing a question that blunted the seriousness of their protest. In one such case of hesitant objection, the interviewee said ''I can't believe you are doing that?" to her friend who was beating to death a possum with a brick. Another interviewee watched as her male friends shot paintballs at birds, squirrels, and cats. She noted: "Once they started like hitting animals I didn't really … I mean like I never told them, I never like said, I was serious about them 'you guys need to stop, this is wrong.' Like I would just joke and be like 'guys, stop, that's not right.' I never really pursued that." A few interviewees were clearer with their criticism, saying things like "leave him alone," "what's wrong with you?" "that wasn't necessary," "why did you do that?" "you shouldn't do that, it's really bad," or "stop," but even these comments often came across hesitantly and without much conviction because they were often posed as questions, were not said sternly, and were not repeated.

Eight percent of the interviewees (2) walked away during the abuse, without saying or doing anything to stop it. In one case, the interviewee left the scene after seeing his friends play "frog baseball" (pitching frogs to a batter to hit) and, in the other case, the interviewee left after a friend choked his pet dog. By silently withdrawing, interviewees forfeited the chance to explain their protest to the abusers who were left in the dark about the symbolic meaning of the interviewees' withdrawal and the extent to which they disapproved of the abuse.

Only twenty percent of the interviewees (5) tried to directly intervene when observing cruelty. Three of these interviewees witnessed chronic animal abuse by parents or cousins who routinely harmed family pets; two of the three felt confident that the abusers would not harm them if they tried to intervene because of their personal knowledge of, and relationships with, the abusers. Two interviewees risked personal harm by physically intervening to stop strangers from harming animals. One interviewee was at a party when she saw a dog urinate on the kitchen floor, after which the dog's owner roughly shoved the dog's face in the urine and then punched the dog several times in its side to the point where the dog could not get up. Although the interviewee purportedly tried to throw herself between the dog and the abuser or perhaps assault him, she was stopped by her friends who feared that the abuser would hurt her too. Another interviewee stopped a dog from being beaten by physically assaulting the abuser, allegedly throwing him to the ground and repeatedly punching him in the face. Moreover, the interviewee claimed that when he decided to assault the abuser, he did not know whether the abuser's friends, who were present, might have attacked him.

Although few interviewees took definitive steps to stop abuse as it unfolded, even less was done to prevent its recurrence. None of the interviewees reported the abuse to any adult authority figure, whether familiar (e.g., parent or teacher) or formal (e.g., police officer or humane law enforcement agent), who might have intervened to speak with, warn, and educate abusers about the inappropriateness, if not criminality, of their acts.

The Barriers

Three general barriers (situational constraints, costs, and personal characteristics) stopped many interviewees from making any intervention or tempered the response of others, consistent with prior research on bystander behavior with human victims. However, the form and salience of these barriers were different, sometimes strikingly so, when bystanders faced animal victims.

Situational Constraints

Research shows that peers' thinking and acting influence how youthful bystanders perceive and behave in jointly occupied situations (Heise 1998; Foubert 2000; Hong 2000; Schwartz et al. 2001; Stein 2007). Most interviewees felt constrained by a definition of animal abuse that made it not criminal, morally reprehensible, or even a lapse in good judgment, but rather a form of roughhousing or "dirty play" (Arluke 2002) engaged in by adolescents outside the purview of adult authority figures. Less commonly, interviewees felt constrained by other situational definitions, including the view that violence toward people and animals is a normal part of everyday life. These definitions drew in interviewees as unwitting and unsupportive accomplices, making them feel anomic—unclear as to how they should behave—sometimes bothered by what they saw, but most times confused about what, if anything, should be done to help the victims or said to the perpetrators and others present.

Dirty Play: Many interviewees found themselves part of a situation that smacked of illicitness and aggressiveness common in the activities of adolescent boys but not limited to harming animals. Like the dirty play of using profanities, telling racist jokes, playing with fire by lighting aerosol sprays or gasoline, or sneaking pornographic photos to look at, the "play" of harming animals seemed to fall into this category of play gone bad from the bystanders' perspective.

According to many interviewees, their former youthful peers perceived violence toward animals as fun, much as middle-school children view violence in general as fun (Kerbs and Jolley 2007). As one interviewee noted, "It was a normal kid's thing. She was kinda like just doing it for fun or something, but at the same time, [it was] dangerous and potentially harmful." Another gave an example of this violent play: "The cat would be runnin' around and he would try to entice him to, you know, play with it, you know, grab it and stuff like that. He would uh, he would just pretty much do anything that you said, like, to the cat, and so, but, um, one of my friends would be like, try to grab him, and, the cat was like petrified of him cause he knew he would, you know, play with him, but play with him to hurt him."

The appearance of play and fun initially led some interviewees to not see abuse, at least until the incidents proceeded to become more demonstratively harmful to the victims. In one case, two boys' "playing" with rats appeared at first to the interviewee and her friends only to be having fun. However, after watching the boys dunk the rat underwater for periods of about half a minute and then seeing the rat in distress, the interviewee and her friends started to question whether this was mere play.

As with other forms of dirty play, most of the reported episodes occurred in the shadows of parents, older siblings, or other authority figures whose absence enabled the mistreatment of animals because no one was present to negatively sanction the untoward behavior. Episodes occurred when parents were away at work or took place in out-of-the-way locations, like along the banks of an unfrequented river. Without sanctioners present, the dirty play became a secret that bystanders now shared.

Unwitting Inclusion: Many interviewees felt that others present during the abuse considered them to be "part of the action." The definition of the situation as dirty play included interviewees as participants rather than observers, even though they opposed the abuse, wanted no part of it, and did nothing overtly to assist or encourage it. This anomic state—being in a role they rejected or were uncomfortable with—confused them and made it difficult to speak out or leave the scene.

Although interviewees did not directly aid the abusers' tormenting, torturing, or killing of animals, they often felt their presence indirectly supported these unseemly behaviors. If they said nothing and were motionless, but stayed as the incidents unfolded, interviewees became part of an audience for abusers to entertain. By using cruelty to get some reaction from others present—including passive bystanders—abusers were seen as "performing" or offering a "show." In the words of one interviewee: "I think they realized we were watching and then it kind of turned into a whole activity … a show. I think they may have been trying to make us laugh. I think, I would say, like, if we had left, the fun probably would've stopped." In fact, many interviewees recalled feeling that the abuse was only performed for their benefit. As one interviewee said of her sister's tormenting of a mouse, "If she was alone, I don't think she would do anything."

A few felt they supported abusers by having some reaction that appeared to be positive or at least not critical, such as surprise or laughter, making the interviewees feel they were almost accomplices. In this vein, one interviewee acknowledged how his laughter might have inadvertently supported the abuser's acts and the definition of the situation as dirty play. He remembered: "I mean I can't say that I had nothing to do with it because I mean I was there. I would get, you know, I would show a reaction after he did it, and you know, he thought that was funny, or he liked it. He would look at me for my reaction, and, bein' 14 years old I would, you know, I would laugh. I was kinda like taken aback but um, you know, I never told him to stop or anything like that."

Because those present perceived interviewees as part of the audience for abuse that at least tacitly approved it, they felt morally responsible for what transpired and members of a club to which they did not want to belong. The fact that interviewees felt they were different from others in terms of their disapproval or discomfort with cruelty gave most of them little emotional or moral comfort in the moment or resolve to behave much differently were they to find themselves in a similar future situation.

Normal Violence: Some interviewees contextualized the abuse they witnessed in ways that normalized it. This normalization presented yet another barrier to interviewees because it made abuse unfortunate but explainable and maybe forgivable.

A couple of interviewees viewed the abuse as a form of discipline, albeit difficult to watch. For example, one interviewee would see his mother slap and kick the family cat for kicking dirt out of a potted plant or eating food left on the kitchen counter. From the perspective of an eight-year-old, his mother was only "disciplining" the cat for its bad behavior. Now, looking back at his mother's treatment of the cat, the interviewee felt that his mother's actions were inappropriate. "When I started getting older, I started to think how could she do that."

Another way for interviewees to normalize abuse was to see it as part of a broader pattern of inevitable, albeit unfortunate, everyday violence toward humans and animals. Some interviewees were accustomed to seeing violence in their neighborhoods and communities. One interviewee was disturbed when he saw his barber use a broomstick handle to repeatedly hit a caged dog, but did nothing because he saw or heard about violence, sometimes much more extreme, on a regular basis that no one stopped, so this dog beating seemed unremarkable. In his words, "Like I've seen animals being treated badly, so it's just like it's almost one of those things like I feel bad, but it's just like I've become so used to that."

Other interviewees normalized abuse because they were used to seeing violence at home, sometimes directed at them. One interviewee, who did not intervene, saw her father kick and beat the family dogs, but was used to him also beating all the children in the family including her. She said: "It was normal to hit your dogs, it was normal to hit your kids. It was just another mean thing my father did. People went hunting and animals were property. I didn't tell anyone because there wasn't anything to tell."

A few interviewees normalized abuse because they saw animals being harmed on television, without anyone stopping it or being punished. In one case, for example, the interviewee, when he was nine years old, often saw his mother hit the family cat with a broom, but decided that it was acceptable for her to do this because he saw similar acts on television cartoons. He said: "Honestly, like the broom thing, I didn't think it [cat beating] was all that bad cause I grew up like watching little things like Tom and Jerry, and Tom and Jerry did the same thing, like Tom getting hit by his owner with a broom, so I was just like, oh."

Costs

Researchers have shown that adult bystanders can be deterred from helping victims if they fear being physically harmed by offenders (Moriarity 1975; Shotland and Straw 1976; Bickman and Helwig 1979; Shotland and Goodstein 1984; Cope, Madfis and Levin 2010) or looking silly by doing the wrong things (Tice and Baumeister 1985). Also, the financial cost of intervening stops many bystanders from helping (Clark and Word 1972; Howard and Crano 1974; Sheleff 1978; Shotland and Stebbins 1983; Bell et al. 1995).

However, most interviewees in this study were concerned about other costs that made them reluctant to intervene. Although some were concerned that reporting abuse would alienate friends, far more common was fear of being embarrassed because intervening was "none of their business" or, even worse, being ridiculed as a "rat." This latter finding supports research that shows the salience of anti-intervention norms during childhood and adolescence (Latane and Rodin 1969; Shotland and Straw 1976; Greenberg et al. 1979; Chekroun and Brauer 2002; Rothe, Elgert and Deedo 2002; O'Campo, Shelley and Jaycox 2007; Cope, Madfis and Levin 2010) and the fear of negative social repercussions if one tries to help victims (Pellegrini 2002; Bauman 2007).

Physical Danger: The vast majority of interviewees did not think they would be physically harmed if they intervened, so this issue did not influence their decision, one way or the other, to say or do something at the time. In most cases when intervention occurred, interviewees felt unthreatened by the abusers because they knew them and felt sure there would be no physical retaliation if they tried to stop the abuse.

In only two cases did fear of physical retaliation pose a serious barrier to intervening. One interviewee softened his criticism so as not to anger the abuser. After seeing a friend choke his pet dog, the interviewee said something to the abuser about doing this, but minced his words, fearing that he would "piss off" his friend in his own home if the objection and protest were direct and stern. In a second case, the interviewee and her siblings frequently saw their father kick and beat the family dog over several years but said nothing to him because they feared being hit themselves were they to question the abuse.

In fact, three interviewees intervened even though they could not rule out being physically harmed. In one case, the interviewee thought the abuser's friends could jump him, but he still intervened because the cruelty (beating a dog) so disturbed him and because he had experience fighting. In the second case, the female interviewee's small size and lack of fighting experience made for no match had a fight occurred with the male abuser, but she acted impulsively because the cruelty (punching a dog) so distressed her, only to be restrained by friends as she lunged toward the abuser. And in the third case, the interviewee risked being harmed by her father who had beaten her before, but she intervened because she, too, was so troubled by the abuse (beating the family dog).

Alienating Friendships: Fear of losing or alienating relationships did not stop most interviewees from intervening. Those without prior relationships with abusers had no relationships to lose or compromise; others felt strongly about stopping the abuse, so losing or alienating relationships did not matter to them; and yet others were confident about their relationships' strength with the abusers, so they did not feel that intervening would seriously affect the quality of these relationships.

In the few cases where relationships deteriorated after interviewees intervened, the change occurred because interviewees distanced themselves from abusers rather than the reverse.

For example, one interviewee saw her cousin kick her pet Chihuahua after it recently had surgery. After telling him to stop and the incident passed, she could not avoid seeing him at family events, but she acted "cool" toward him at future meetings. In another case, after the interviewee saw his friend choke a dog, he told him this was wrong and let the friendship lapse over time.

However, some interviewees told abusers they did not like their behavior, but failed to report the incidents to authority figures or owners of the abused animals because they feared doing this might jeopardize their relationships with the abusers or lead to unwelcomed repercussions. For example, one interviewee was afraid that her sister would get mad at her if their mother were told about the incident (mouse being spray painted), so she said nothing to her mother. In these cases, interviewees reflected that possible damage to their friendships weighed more heavily on them than the extent of animal suffering they perceived, at the time of the incident.

Awkwardness: A cost that deterred more interviewees was the anticipated awkwardness of being told that intervening was "none of their business." Bystanders who witness violence between family members sometimes see this untoward behavior as a "family" issue (Heise 1998; Fox 1999) and do not intervene. In a few cases, interviewees felt it was inappropriate to say or do anything about the abuse they witnessed because they saw the abuse as an issue between the owner and his or her pet, much like the situation people find themselves in when they see a parent harshly scold a child and feel that it is none of their business to say anything.

The public etiquette to mind one's own business became a barrier to some interviewees even when the abuser was not a complete stranger. For example, the interviewee who observed his long-time barber forcefully hit his own pet dog with a pole said that not having a close relationship with the barber made it difficult for him to say anything about the dog's mistreatment. Although the interviewee's barber was not a complete stranger, apparently their relationship's formality and impersonality presented a barrier to intervening. Compounding his silence, the interviewee added that there were other men present in the barbershop who were applauding the abuser's behavior, making it all the more difficult for him to do anything. He said: "I felt like it wasn't really my place to say anything, you know. It's like it's a more public setting. It's just, it's not your place to do anything. You can't really say anything."

Etiquette even became a barrier in a few cases when the abuser was a close friend or a close friend's companion. In one case, for example, the interviewee saw a good friend's boyfriend roughly grab and throw several dogs over the side of a bridge into a river fifteen feet below. The interviewee considered saying something but did not because she felt it was wrong to do so, under the circumstances, since she had not seen her friend for a long time and was there to rebuild their friendship and to meet the new boyfriend.

Teasing: The most commonly reported cost of intervening was the fear of being labeled a "rat," "tattletale," "backstabber," or "spoilsport." In a typical case, the interviewee, who watched two boys dunk a rat in a can of water to drown it, said, when asked if she considered telling the boys' parents: "We were going to, we were about to, in my head I remember, but in my head we didn't want to be tattletales, you know at that age." Another interviewee thought that reporting the abuse (body-slamming a dog) to the pet's owner—the abuser's girlfriend—might cost him his friendship with the abuser. "I was really afraid like if I told her, like, what would that make me, would he consider me as a friend? It's like if I were to tell her, like, so he would've viewed me as like a traitor, or like as a backstabber or something like that extreme."

In some cases, interviewees went to great lengths to avoid these negative labels. One interviewee left the scene of abuse (frog crushing) as soon as it started and randomly rode his bike for almost two hours, fearing that if he came home early from this play date his mother would ask him why and then call the abuser's mother to tell her what happened. Had she made this call, the interviewee felt certain that his friends would have labeled him a "rat."

If not belittled as a rat or tattletale, some interviewees were worried about being teased or given a hard time by their friends for spoiling the fun of dirty play. One interviewee reflected: "I think, cause of my age, um, you know, that middle-school age, I wanted, I didn't want to be the one that took away from the, took away from the fun, you know, like I didn't want to be 'Stop doing that!' and you know I feel like the other two kids would look at me and be like, 'yo, what's wrong with you,' so I just kept my, you know, I just kept it under the radar and just let it be." Another interviewee had a sister put paint and nail polish on a captured mouse. Although seeing this bothered the interviewee when the nail polish got in the mouse's eyes and it started to squeak, she did not say anything to her sister because "I just wouldn't want her to think of me as like a wimp." And yet another interviewee explained that she felt like a "downer" for breaking the dirty-play definition of abuse:

> I felt really bad about taking it, like, away, like on one hand I was worried for my guinea pig and it was like, mine, but then on the other hand, I felt really bad like kinda like defying my cousin. He was like "you're ruining the fun … why are you getting all upset about it for no reason?" And I was like, distressed. I kinda like was torn about it and felt bad about it but I did it anyways despite the conflict. I felt bad about saving my guinea pig cause um I was like not cool [laughs]. I was being a downer. Like I felt really like I was taking away their toy, and I felt bad about it, but I have such empathy for animals.

Some of the teasing for spoiling dirty play was gendered. In one case, a female interviewee was reluctant to criticize a male who was beating to death a possum because "He probably would've just been like 'oh, you're just being a girl and feeling bad for things, who cares.'" Another female interviewee felt uneasy about fulfilling gendered expectations because rescuing the victimized animal would be seen as an "emotional overreaction." She said: "I was like an emotional girl about it. I felt like I was overreacting. It was a boy who was doing it and then like I was like 'being a girl.' It was like worse that I was protect … I dunno, it was kinda like, halfway okay that I was doing it because I was a girl, so I was allowed to be more emotional and weaker about it, and like not as gung-ho, but on the other hand, it's like you're like playing too. You're either like trying to be a boy, or you're being a weak girl, I dunno."

Personal Characteristics

Some research indicates that individual qualities stemming from the bystander's demographic background, sense of efficacy, ability, and knowledge of what to do (Huston et al. 1981; Rothe, Elgert and Deedo 2002; Banyard, Plante and Moynihan 2004, 2007), social network (Amato 1990), or compassion (Dovidio 1984) can influence whether human victims of violence or emergencies are helped. In different ways, personal characteristics influenced whether adolescent bystanders intervened to help animal victims.

Gender and Age: Certain demographic components, particularly gender and age, appeared to influence interviewees' response to abuse. When comparing all interveners with all non-interveners, gender seemed unimportant. However, when only looking at interviewees who directly responded in physical ways to stop abuse, males appeared much less likely to take action. This finding is consistent with research showing that females are more likely to intervene than male bystanders (Salmivalli, Kaukiainen and Lagerspetz 1998; Burn 2009) either because male bystanders receive vicarious gratification from seeing a weaker victim being harmed (Borofsky, Stollak and Messé 1971) or because they feel that intervening will make them look weak (Carlson 2008). Given the small number of respondents, further scrutiny of this pattern is necessary.

Gender also influenced bystander behavior in another way: while it operated to deter intervention for both sexes, it did so in different ways. Some females reflected on how the indirectness or hesitancy of their objections led male abusers to disregard them. For example the interviewee who observed her male roommate using a brick to beat to death a possum, felt that her objection—"Why are you doing that?"—appeared even milder because she was a female. She said: "I'm not sure that he realized that I meant it … that it's not just being sympathetic or acting like a girl. That it was mean, and not necessary. Instead he just laughs it off, like you're, 'please, you're just …'" While some female interviewees felt confined by their gender roles to express their objections obliquely, some male interviewees felt pressure, as peers to the male abusers, to go along with the abuse and say nothing.

Indeed, the definition of abuse as a form of dirty play that interviewees stumbled upon was itself a gendered activity—it was something that young males typically did for fun and that young girls found distressing. As one upset college-aged female said about a friend who was throwing a cat down the stairs, "He kinda laughed, cause I think he just figured it was like a boy thing to do. Like, cause he's a boy, it's ok for him to be aggressive towards it and stuff. And like it was just a joke, and ha ha." Another interviewee said that even gossiping about the abuse with classmates was itself a gendered activity, limited to sharing among boys: "In the middle school people would tell the story and you'd get completely different reactions from some kids. Some kids would just laugh, like 'you're crazy' um, 'man, that's nuts' and then, I remember like, we never told any girls, that was the other thing, I specifically remember, because their reaction would be much different, it was all guys." When bystanders were female and abusers were male, gender role expectations often played out in ways that supported this definition of the situation and stifled concerted criticism. Adolescent female bystanders often felt that gender disadvantaged them because their criticism of the abuser's acts would be trivialized by males present as overly sympathetic and emotional, given the adolescent male view of the victims as "only animals" and of the displays of aggression as highly valued. From the female bystander's perspective, then, the male abuser's playful, roughhousing attitude trumped any dissent, especially since males present usually outnumbered the female's lone voice.

The bystander's age also seemed to influence whether and how interviewees responded. Age distinguished interveners from non-interveners; interveners were generally older than non-interveners, a finding inconsistent with research on children defending victimized peers that says such intervening is less common as children age (Salmivalli 1999; Henderson and Hymel 2002; Menesini, Codecasa and Benelli 2003). One interviewee illustrated this difference, having intervened to stop friends from throwing rocks at squirrels when he was a late teenager, but not intervening at eight when his friend threw the family kitten down a two-story laundry shoot. While he did not like seeing the squirrels wince in pain after being hit by stones, the idea of the kitten being hurt from the fall did not seem to register on his youthful sensibilities as something that was wrong and should not be done. He reflected: "I feel, in 3rd grade I really didn't even think past that. Yeah. I didn't … I dunno, it seemed almost like a cool idea for me to do, I was like, oh I want to do this! I wanna go down the laundry shoot."

There also were some age differences among interviewees who did not intervene. Certain responses or rationales for not responding were more typical for younger than for older bystanders, according to the respondents' recollections. Younger bystanders were more likely to say that their apathy resulted from being unsure how much or whether animal victims suffered, while older bystanders were more likely to explain their apathy by citing the constraints of situational norms and their powerlessness to stop abuse or prevent its recurrence.

Not Being an Animal Person: Intervention seemed less likely among interviewees not having had a special pet connection or a self-concept of an animal person. Pet ownership per se did not distinguish interveners from non-interveners, since almost all interviewees owned pets at one time or another. However, the role, significance, and meaning of pets distinguished many interveners from non-interveners in ways reminiscent of Arluke's (2003) youthful "super-nurturers." Interveners were more likely to have had one or more pets that played a significant role in the family and to have felt a special responsibility for protecting their pets and animals in general. For example, one interviewee who did not intervene to help a ferret that was starved to death and run on an exercise wheel until it was injured or collapsed said that not having a pet herself may have played a role in her passivity, saying, "I didn't have pets at this time, yeah. So that's why I think I didn't really understand the severity of it because I didn't have pets at home. I didn't know."

Also related to pets, interveners as opposed to non-interveners were more likely to see wild, low status animal victims as pet-like—resembling their own or someone else's pet, or having their own animal families—thereby inspiring intervention. In one case, the interviewee spoke out to stop the stoning of a wild rabbit because she had a pet rabbit and did not want someone to do that to her pet. Conversely, not being able to see a victim as pet-like usually stopped intervention. This was the case with one interviewee who, because she could not see an abused rat as pet-like, watched passively as it was poked to death with a stick.

Interveners more likely recalled an internal moral conviction, often but not always related to being an "animal person," that compelled them to tell those present during the abuse that their acts were wrong, even if the interviewee's words would do nothing to stop the abuser's actions then or in the future. As one interviewee said of his reaction, "I've been raised, and just thought, myself, that it's completely wrong to do anything like that, so I had to say something."

Interveners articulated this moral obligation in different ways. Some spoke about the triggering of a feeling that made them think that harming animals was wrong. Unable to clearly define this inner state, sometimes calling it a "gut feeling," they acknowledged, in so many words, that at the time of the abuse they had not yet formed a consciousness or moral perspective that extended to the mistreatment of animals, but, nevertheless, sensed the injustice and gratuitousness of what they saw. One interviewee, for example, remembered being confused about seeing his mother beat the family cat, but feeling, at the same time, that doing this to the cat was wrong. "The fact that like deep down it's like I'm still young and don't really have like clear set ways of thinking but deep down I knew it was wrong."

Other interveners said that this moral obligation stemmed from being an "animal lover." They spoke about being taught to respect animals and to see cruelty as wrong, having had parents who rescued animals, and always having had an eye out for animals in distress who they would help. To explain her intervention, one interviewee said that she intervened not just because the victim was her pet and might have had its legs broken from the abuse, but because she felt "responsible" for its care, saying "I like really really, I loved animals a lot. Like I would be the kid who would just like lie on the ground and watch the cat so it didn't run away."

And other interveners felt that this moral obligation stemmed from their sense of themselves as defenders of people who were being bullied or were helpless as well as animals that were victimized. These interveners felt that doing nothing in such situations made them responsible for whatever harm transpired to victims, and that even if intervening failed it was important to take a moral stand by protesting. To wit, one interviewee recalled his conversion from being a passive bystander to an intervener after seeing a friend bullied at school and having been taught by one of his teachers "you're just as bad if you're watching it happen."

Reconciling Abuse: Also deterring intervention, interviewees sometimes tried to reduce the dissonance of seeing close friends or family members harm animals by excusing or justifying their behavior. These excuses and justifications made it difficult for interviewees to say or do anything to stop or prevent abuse because this thinking exceptionalized or normalized the abuse.

Interviewees often recalled seeing abusers as "good hearted," nonviolent, or perhaps troubled but not "bad." For example, one interviewee chose to ignore her mother's abuse of the family cat because, otherwise, the mother seemed to care for and be attached to the victim; she even paid $1400 for the cat to have emergency surgery, despite the family's meager working-class income. Other interviewees pointed out that the abusers would never hurt or bully humans, to indicate that they were not generally violent or dangerous to people or presumably to animals. As one interviewee said of his abuser friend: "Good hearted kid … he wasn't a bully, he wasn't mean, he was just, he was out to entertain people and anyone that he could get a rise out of, or wanna hang out with him more, would you know, increase his popularity. He would do some pretty crazy things." If not basically a good person, some interviewees excused the abusers as troubled people as opposed to bad persons. An example of this excuse was given by an interviewee who saw her friends torture and starve their pet ferret: "I don't see them, I don't see them as being mean people, I just see them as being kind of like, lost."

Other interviewees excused their friends' abuse by focusing on situational pressures beyond their control. For example, one interviewee felt that his abuser friend liked the animal victim but harmed it because he caved into pressure to perform for his friends by hurting the animal. "He wasn't like a, uh, cold-hearted by no means. So, I don't think he was doin' it, you know, on his own, just purposefully tryin' to injure the cat, because I feel like he liked it. But people were watching and said 'do it,' you know what I mean." Another interviewee thought that his friend's abuse of a dog departed from his normal unaggressive behavior, concluding that the abuse must have been due to the stressful relationship he had with his girlfriend who owned the dog. He said, "He would never do this to a person. I've never seen him be like … I don't know. It's this relationship that's causing him to take it out on her, that's what I think."

And a few interviewees justified the abuse by blaming the victim. One interviewee blamed the cat for causing the abuser to have bad allergic attacks that incensed the cat owner and made her take out her own suffering on the animal. Another interviewee blamed the family cat for constantly ripping apart the garbage can in the kitchen, making her mother understandably very frustrated and angry toward the victimized animal.

Feeling Ineffective: Several interviewees felt uncomfortable intervening, doing little or nothing to stop or prevent abuse, because they had no confidence in their ability to do so. In one case, an interviewee who saw her roommate beat to death a possum only said to the abuser, "Why are you doing that?" When asked why she was not more forceful, she replied: "I didn't know what to do, how to go about it. And I don't think I have really any authority so he [abuser] would probably be like 'go away.'" In two cases, interviewees spoke about not feeling physically confident enough to intervene. For example, one interviewee for years saw his mother kick, smack, and stomp on their family cat, but said nothing to her because he did not feel strong enough to stand up to and criticize her. He only stood up for the abused cat after he started playing sports and feeling stronger, which gave him newfound confidence in his ability to protect people and animals.

More commonly, interviewees were pessimistic about stopping what they witnessed or preventing future abuse. They felt that nothing would stop abusers from harming animals when they were present, short of a parent coming upon the scene of abuse unexpectedly, and even the latter (see below) was often seen dubiously. One interviewee had hoped that the abusers might have momentarily stopped their cruelty out of "respect" to him while he was present, only to be disappointed. "I knew that they wouldn't stop because that was just the kind of kids that they were. But since I was there, I was hoping they would give me that respect at least, but they didn't at all. They were rather selfish most of the time that I dealt with them, and this was no exception."

Interviewees were uniformly pessimistic about being able to change the abuser's behavior in the future. One interviewee who, after he saw his friend slam a dog to the floor, told the abuser that doing this was wrong. When the same abuse happened two or three times in the following weeks the interviewee again told his friend that he should stop doing this. In subsequent weeks, he heard from other friends that the abuse continued unabated, but decided to not speak to the abuser because it was useless. He said, "I don't know, like, I don't think he'd listen to me because apparently like similar situations, like cruelty, like keep happening."

Feeling Alone: Research shows that having friends present who encourage intervention increases the likelihood of helping behavior (Latane and Darley 1968; Latane and Rodin 1969; Greenberg et al. 1979). In the present study, humane allies were on the scene in only a few cases, either supporting the interviewee's intervention, leading the way for it, or continuing it after the fact. In one case, an 18-year-old male interviewee and his brother watched a friend throw a cat out a three-story window. The interviewee said that he was quick to tell the abuser "Hey stop, this is stupid" because his brother immediately "jumped all over" the abuser and "rubbed in" how wrong it was to treat the cat this way.

More typically, interviewees felt like they alone were upset and critical of the abuser's actions, having no humane allies present to support their intervention or lead the way; this feeling deterred most from taking bolder steps to stop or prevent abuse. Some interviewees did not have any humane allies present because they were truly alone—either they were the only ones with the abusers or others present were also harming animals or clearly supporting it. When there were other bystanders present, most interviewees assumed that fellow onlookers did not share their opposition to the abuse but were instead indifferent to, or entertained by, the abuser. Sometimes they felt convinced of this because others present seemed to enjoy or even encourage the abuser's behavior. In either case, interviewees did not consider the possibility that fellow bystanders felt pressured to behave this way and may in fact have been as distressed as they were by the abuse.

Interviewees' sense of isolation also stemmed from the belief that they could not count on adults to support their interventions. Most thought that adults were unavailable because they worked far from the scene of the cruelty, thereby preventing them from supporting the interviewees in a timely fashion. Although interviewees could still have reported the incidents to parents or others, they did not because they feared being labeled as "tattle tales" or getting the abusers and themselves punished. One interviewee, whose guinea pig was being abused by her cousins, did not consider telling her parents because "Usually my cousins and siblings, we usually decided things among ourselves, cause my parents usually punished everyone. So it was better to try to deal with it ourselves." And other interviewees did not report the abuse to parents or other adult authority figures because they felt that doing so would be useless. The interviewee who saw her roommate beat to death a possum said: "If it [abuse] was brought up, he [abuser's father] probably would've just like laughed it off and they [parents] would've just like from my own experience with parents, they probably would've just been like 'I can't believe you did that' but nothing huge." Indeed, many interviewees thought their parents did not regard animal abuse to be a bad thing, or were at least unsure of their reaction; to wit, one interviewee said of her parents: "I mean nothing against my parents, but they aren't like 'animal cruelty is bad.' They would never really say anything."

The feeling of being alone, without support, extended to peers, real or imagined. In one case, the interviewee did not get support from friends at school when they heard about the incident, saying "No one ever called him [the abuser] out on it enough to be like, you know 'You're a bad person.' It would just be kinda like 'Oh, that's kinda weird' or 'That's crazy, it's awesome! I gotta see that,' you know." In a few cases, interviewees said that had peers been present during the abuse, they would not have served as humane allies. For example, one interviewee who was alone when seeing his friend throw a dog against a wall, and who heard subsequent reports from his abusing friend about mistreating this dog, believed that had others been present they would have applauded the abuser's efforts and served as "accomplices" to the abuse, leaving the interviewee by himself to protest his friend's acts.

And even if present, having humane allies did not ensure that interviewees spoke out, left the scene, or physically intervened to stop the abuse. In one case, for example, the interviewee, along with her friend, witnessed repeated attempts to drown a rat, leading to its slow death. This bystander did not speak out or otherwise intervene, despite the presence of her friend who was more upset than the interviewee about the rat's cruel treatment.

Discussion

Results of this study suggest that many child and adolescent bystanders of animal abuse face barriers to intervening that resemble, in general terms, the barriers faced by bystanders of violence against humans. These common barriers stem from situational constraints, perceived costs, and personal characteristics that deter intervention. However, when examined closely, the nature and salience of these barriers appear to be expressed differently for youthful bystanders of animal abuse. For example, situational constraints, such as the pressure to see animal abuse as dirty play, perceived costs, such as the fear of being labeled a tattletale, and personal characteristics, such as a sense of isolation, appeared to be important deterrents to intervention for young bystanders of animal abuse but not for adult bystanders of human violence.

These results have practical and policy applications. Educators, advocates, and policy makers interested in developing and promoting antiviolence programs for children and adolescents desperately need information about the sources of bystander apathy in cases of animal cruelty. Bystander empowerment programs are expanding their work with teens to raise consciousness and enhance helping behavior toward all victims of violence, whether human or animal, but lack the empirical information needed to construct realistic teaching scenarios of bystander apathy in cruelty cases or to more generally coach and advise children and adolescents about how to intervene in these situations. Social science research, such as that reported here, can play a vital role in this regard by providing detailed, empirically based information about the kinds of barriers faced by youthful bystanders of cruelty.

Although most interviewees did little to stop or prevent what they witnessed, other than showing some hesitant and ambiguous resistance, results suggest that many of these interviewees were not humanely indifferent to the abuse. To some degree, their hesitancy to respond could reflect, in part, the ambiguous and conflicting attitudes our society holds towards animals (Arluke and Sanders 1996). Nevertheless, it was clear that many interviewees were troubled by the abuse, wanted it to end, and hoped it would not be repeated in the future, but felt unable or ill equipped to do anything to change what they saw or what might happen again, other than avoiding the abusers. Rather, they were engulfed by situational constraints often fraught with ambiguous, complicated, and even risky choices that unfolded without warning and ended quickly.

This suggests that humane education programs aimed at teaching children and adolescents about the needs of animals and instilling prosocial attitudes toward animals, such as empathy, might be misdirected if not redundant. A more effective strategy might be to design and target interventions aimed at empowering bystander behavior in situations where children and adolescents encounter untoward behavior toward animals. There is empirical support for reducing animal abuse by improving bystander responses. For example, programs have successfully empowered bystanders to prevent sexual violence on college campuses (Banyard, Moynihan and Crossman 2009), suggesting that such an approach could be a useful way to attack the underlying sense of inefficacy and pessimism felt by bystanders of animal violence.

More specifically, knowledge and strategies about how to intervene need to be addressed, since many interviewees had no idea what to do when witnessing animal cruelty. Research suggests that if potential bystanders are trained in emergency aid or given options as to how they would help in general situations, they report being more comfortable with intervening (Rothe, Elgert and Deedo 2002; Banyard, Plante and Moynihan 2004, 2007).

Use of such knowledge and strategies might be particularly effective and safe when bystanders observe abuse by friends and family rather than strangers. With most interviewees, the abusers were not strangers who represented unknown strength or danger if the interviewees intervened directly. Rather, they were often long-term friends, siblings, or parents with whom the interviewees felt completely unthreatened physically because they had an established pattern of interacting with the abusers that was safe and predictable. Yet most interviewees still either did nothing or only spoke out, often hesitantly. The few exceptions stood out. For example, one interviewee removed a cat from the abuser's reach that stopped this abuse from repeating most of the time. In cases where the offender's motive is simply boredom, or a "hobby," having alternative ideas of things to do, or distractions, may be all it takes to reduce the number of incidences, if not extinguish them entirely. In one case, for example, the interviewee suggested to his friend who was hitting squirrels with rocks that he might enjoy playing basketball, which worked to distract him from the rock-throwing preoccupation to a different form of "recreation." Obviously, this strategy would not be effective in cases where the intent is malicious, or the offender is pursuing violence much more doggedly, but in cases of boredom it could work.

Bystander training can also address some of the costs of intervening in animal cruelty cases. Since the primary cost found in this study was fear of being labeled a tattletale or spoilsport, programs should be designed to help potential bystanders deal with such negative appraisal. For example, cognitive-behavioral techniques could be used to make adolescents more equipped to manage this concern, should they find themselves in a position to possibly intervene to help an animal. Such techniques could involve exercises to identify and challenge negative ways of thinking and to replace these with more positive thought patterns (Turk, Heimberg and Hope 2001; Andrews et al. 2003). Although researchers have not examined whether prospective techniques increase the likelihood of intervention by youthful bystanders of animal abuse, a few studies have shown that cognitive-behavioral techniques can enhance the likelihood of bystander intervention with human victims.

Finally, in addition to having practical and policy implications, the exploratory nature of this study's findings call for further clarification and verification of the sources of bystander apathy in animal abuse cases and their salience to children and adolescents. To do this, researchers would do well to expand the demographic composition of their samples to include a more economically and cultural diverse study population than was obtained in the present study. Researchers also should ask the flip question, long neglected in the existing literature on bystander behavior with human victims (Manning, Levine and Collins 2007): why do some bystanders make an effort to help victims? Although this study found that child and adolescent bystanders faced substantial barriers that stopped or limited their interventions to help or protect animal victims, a few interviewees did make clear-cut attempts to stop animal abuse. In this regard, researchers might examine how personal characteristics of bystanders, such as pet ownership or identity as "animal people," appear to override the situational constraints presented by adolescent peer culture to not intervene.

Acknowledgements

This research was supported by a grant from A Kinder World Foundation. I am grateful to Kathy Savesky for her encouragement and support.

References

Amato, P. 1990. Personality and social network involvement as predictors of helping behavior in everyday life. *Social Psychology Quarterly* 53: 31–43.

Andrews, G., Creamer, M., Crino, R., Hunt, C., Lampe, L. and Page, A. 2003. *The Treatment of Anxiety Disorders: Clinician Guides and Patient Manuals*. 2nd edn. Cambridge: Cambridge University Press.

Arluke, A. 2002. Animal abuse as dirty play. *Symbolic Interaction* 25: 405–430.

Arluke, A. 2003. The childhood origins of supernurturance: The social context of early humane behavior. *Anthrozoös* 16: 3–27.

Arluke, A. and Sanders, C. 1996. *Regarding Animals*. Philadelphia, PA: Temple University Press.

Banyard, V., Moynihan, M. and Crossman, M. 2009. Reducing sexual violence on campus: The role of student leaders as empowered bystanders. *Journal of College Student Development* 50: 446–457.

Banyard, V., Plante, E. and Moynihan, M. 2004. Bystander education: Bringing a broader community perspective to sexual violence prevention. *Journal of Community Psychology* 32: 61–79.

Banyard, V., Plante, E. and Moynihan, M. 2007. Sexual violence prevention through bystander education: An experimental evaluation. *Journal of Community Psychology* 35: 463–481.

Bauman, S. 2007. Cyberbullying: A virtual menace. Ph.D. Dissertation. Melbourne, Australia.

Bell, J., Grekul, J., Lamba, N., Minas, C. and Harrell, W. 1995. The impact of cost on student helping behavior. *Journal of Social Psychology* 135: 49–56.

Bickman, L. and Helwig, H. 1979. Bystander reporting of a crime: The impact of incentives. *Criminology* 17: 283–300.

Borofsky, G., Stollak, G. and Messé, L. 1971. Sex differences in bystander reactions to physical assault. *Journal of Experimental Social Psychology* 7: 313–318.

Burn, S. 2009. A situational model of sexual assault prevention through bystander intervention. *Sex Roles* 60: 779–792.

Carlson, M. 2008. I'd rather go along and be considered a man: Masculinity and bystander intervention. *The Journal of Men's Studies* 16: 3–17.

Chekroun, P. and Brauer, M. 2002. The bystander effect and social control behavior: The effect of the presence of others on people's reactions to norm violations. *European Journal of Social Psychology* 32: 853–867.

Christianson, S., Goodman, J. and Loftus, E. 1992. Eyewitness memory for stressful events: Methodological quandaries and ethical dilemmas. In *The Handbook of Emotion and Memory*, 217–241, ed. S. Christianson. Hillsdale, NJ: Lawrence Erlbaum.

Clark, R. and Word, L. 1972. Why don't bystanders help? Because of ambiguity? *Journal of Personality and Social Psychology* 24: 392–400.

Cope, S., Madfis, E. and Levin, J. 2010. How gender, anonymity, and social norms affect bystander willingness to intervene. Paper presented at the annual meeting of the American Sociological Association, Atlanta, GA, August 14, 2010.

Costanzo, P. and Shaw, M. 1966. Conformity as a function of age level. *Child Development* 37: 967–975.

Daly, B. and Morton, L. 2003. Children with pets do not show higher empathy: A challenge to current views. *Anthrozoös* 16: 298–314.

Dovidio, J. 1984. Helping behavior and altruism: An empirical and conceptual overview. *Advances in Experimental Social Psychology* 17: 361–414.

Espelage, D., Holt, M. and Henkel, R. 2003. Examination of peer-group contextual effects on aggression during early adolescence. *Child Development* 74: 205–220.

Foubert, J. 2000. The longitudinal effects of a rape-prevention program on fraternity men's attitudes, behavioral intent, and behavior. *Journal of American College Health* 48: 158–163.

Fox, K. 1999. Changing violent minds: Discursive correction and resistance in the cognitive treatment of violent offenders in prison. *Social Problems* 46: 88–103.

Greenberg, M., Wilson, C., Ruback, R. and Mills, M. 1979. The social and emotional determinants of victim crime reporting. *Social Psychology Quarterly* 42: 364–372.

Heise, L. 1998. Violence against women: An integrated, ecological framework. *Violence Against Women* 4: 262–290.

Henderson, N. and Hymel, S. 2002. Peer contributions to bullying in schools: Examining student response categories. Poster presented at the National Association of School Psychologists Annual Convention, Chicago, February, 2002.

Heuer, F. and Reiberg, D. 1992. Emotion, arousal, and memory for detail. In *The Handbook of Emotion and Memory,* 151–180, ed. S. Christianson. Hillsdale, NJ: Lawrence Erlbaum.

Hong, L. 2000. Toward a transformed approach to prevention: Breaking the link between masculinity and violence. *Journal of American College Health* 48: 269–279.

Howard, W. and Crano, W. 1974. Effects of sex, conversation, location, and size of observer group on bystander intervention in a high risk situation. *Sociometry* 37: 491–507.

Huston, T., Ruggiero, M., Conner, R. and Geis, G. 1981. Bystander intervention into crime: A study based on naturally occurring episodes. *Social Psychology Quarterly* 44: 14–23.

Kerbs, J. and Jolley, J. 2007. The joy of violence: What about violence is fun in middle-school? *American Journal of Criminal Justice* 32: 12–29.

Kolbo, J., Blakely, E. and Engleman, D. 1996. Children who witness domestic violence: A review of empirical literature. *Journal of Interpersonal Violence* 11: 281–293.

Latane, B. and Darley, J. 1968. Group inhibition of bystander intervention in emergencies. *Journal of Personality and Social Psychology* 10: 215–221.

Latane, B. and Rodin, J. 1969. A lady in distress: Inhibiting effects of friends and strangers on bystander intervention. *Journal of Experimental Social Psychology* 5: 189–202.

Manning, R., Levine, M. and Collins, A. 2007. The Kitty Genovese murder and the social psychology of helping: The parable of the 38 witnesses. *American Psychologist* 62: 555–562.

Menesini, E., Codecasa, E. and Benelli, B. 2003. Enhancing children's responsibility to take action against bullying: Evaluation of a befriending intervention in Italian middle schools. *Aggressive Behavior* 29: 10–14.

Milgram, S. 1974. *Obedience to Authority.* New York: Harper Collins.

Moriarity, T. 1975. Crime, commitment, and the responsive bystanders: Two field experiments. *Journal of Personality and Social Psychology* 31: 370–376.

O'Campo, B., Shelley, G. and Jaycox, L. 2007. Latino teens talk about help seeking and help giving in relation to dating violence. *Violence Against Women* 13: 172–189.

Pellegrini, A. 2002. Bullying, victimization, and sexual harassment during the transition to middle school. *Educational Psychologist* 37: 151–163.

Piliavin, J., Dovidio, J., Gaertner, S. and Clark, R. 1981. *Emergency Intervention.* New York: Academic.

Rabow, J. Newcomb, M., Monto, M. and Hernandez, A. 1990. Altruism in drunk driving situations: Personal and situational factors in intervention. *Social Psychology Quarterly* 53: 199–213.

Rigby, K. and Johnson, B. 2006. Expressed readiness of Australian schoolchildren to act as bystanders in support of children who are being bullied. *Educational Psychology* 26: 425–440.

Rothe, P., Elgert, L. and Deedo, R. 2002. Dynamic influences on bystander actions: Program recommendations from the field. Alberta Centre for Injury Control and Research, Department of Public Health Sciences, University of Alberta.

Salmivalli, C. 1999. Participant role approach to school bullying: Implications for interventions. *Journal of Adolescence* 22: 453–459.

Salmivalli, C., Kaukiainen, A. and Lagerspetz, K. 1998. Aggression in the social relations of school-aged girls and boys. In *Children's Peer Relations,* 60–75, ed. P. Slee and K. Rigby. London: Routledge.

Schwartz, S. 1977. Normative influences on altruism. *Advances in Experimental Social Psychology* 10: 221–276.

Schwartz, M., DeKeseredy, W., Tait, D. and Alvi, S. 2001. Male peer support and a feminist routine activities theory: Understanding sexual assault on the college campus. *Justice Quarterly* 16: 623–649.

Sheleff, L. 1978. *The Bystander: Behavior, Law, Ethics.* Lexington, MA: Lexington Books.

Shotland, R. and Goodstein, L. 1984. The role of bystanders in crime control. *Journal of Social Issues* 40: 9–26.

Shotland, R. and Stebbins, C. 1983. Emergency and cost as determinants of helping behavior and the slow accumulation of social psychological knowledge. *Social Psychology Quarterly* 46: 36–46.

Shotland, R. and Straw, M. 1976. Bystander response to an assault: When a man attacks a woman. *Journal of Personality and Social Psychology* 34: 990–999.

Stein, J. 2007. Peer educators and close friends as predictors of male college students' willingness to prevent rape. *Journal of College Student Development* 48: 75–89.

Tice, D. and Baumeister, R. 1985. Masculinity inhibits helping in emergencies: Personality does predict the bystander effect. *Personality and Social Psychology* 49: 420–428.

Towns, D. 1996. "Rewind the world!" An ethnographic study of inner-city African American children's perceptions of violence. *Journal of Negro Education* 65: 375–389.

Turk, C., Heimberg, R. and Hope, D. 2001. Social anxiety disorder. In *Clinical Handbook of Psychological Disorders: A Step-By-Step Treatment Manual,* 114–153, ed. D. H. Barlow. New York: Guilford.

Warner, B. and Weist, M. 1996. Urban youth as witnesses to violence: Beginning assessment and treatment efforts. *Journal of Youth and Adolescence* 25: 361–377.

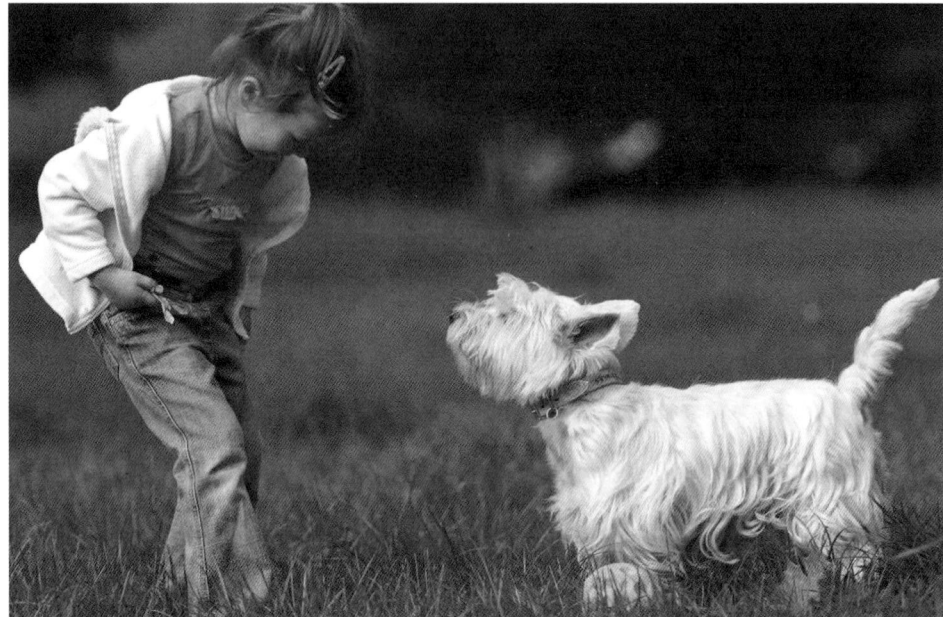

NICHD, WALTHAM® Research Funding Announced

For the past three years, the Eunice Kennedy Shriver National Institute of Child Health and Human Development (NICHD) at the National Institutes of Health and the WALTHAM® Centre for Pet Nutrition, a division of Mars, Inc., have been engaged in a public-private partnership to study the interaction between humans and animals. The partnership encourages human-animal interaction (HAI) research, especially as it relates to child development, health, and the therapeutic use of animals with children and adolescents.

The research awards announced by the partnership earlier this year include funding for the following studies:

- Animal-Assisted Intervention for Children with Autism Spectrum Disorder
  Alan M. Beck, Purdue University West Lafayette
- Dog Presence and Childrens' Stress During Forensic Interviews for Child Abuse
  Rebecca Ann Johnson, University of Missouri-Columbia
- Buffering Role of Pet Dogs on Children's HPA Stress Responses
  Darlene A. Kertes et al., University of Florida
- Impact of Pet Ownership on SA/MRSA Colonization in Children and Families
  Timothy F. Landers et al., Ohio State University
- Characterizing Pet Experience In Infancy and The Relation to Cognitive Development
  Lisa Oakes, University of California Davis

To get more information about this research, visit ***http://projectreporter.nih.gov*** and enter "RFA-HD-12-105" in the FOA field.

*For the latest research, news, funding opportunities and events, register for the WALTHAM® Human-Animal Interaction Newsletter. To subscribe, contact **info@WALTHAMe-newsletter.com**.*

WALTHAM® – Bringing the science to life™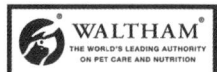

ANTHROZOÖS   VOLUME 25, ISSUE 1   REPRINTS AVAILABLE   PHOTOCOPYING   © ISAZ 2012
PP. 25–34   DIRECTLY FROM   PERMITTED   PRINTED IN THE UK
THE PUBLISHERS   BY LICENSE ONLY

Effects of Presence of a Familiar Pet Dog on Regional Cerebral Activity in Healthy Volunteers: A Positron Emission Tomography Study

Akihiro Sugawara[*], Mohammad Mehedi Masud[*], Akimitsu Yokoyama[†], Wataru Mizutani[‡], Shoichi Watanuki[*], Kazuhiko Yanai[*], Masatoshi Itoh[*] and Manabu Tashiro[*]

*Division of Cyclotron Nuclear Medicine, Cyclotron Radioisotope Center, Tohoku University, Sendai, Japan
†Teikyo University of Science and Technology, Tokyo, Japan
‡Japanese Animal Hospital Association, Tokyo, Japan

Address for correspondence:
Manabu Tashiro, M.D., Ph.D.,
Division of Cyclotron Nuclear
Medicine, Cyclotron and
Radioisotope Center,
Tohoku University,
6-3 Aoba, Aramaki, Aoba-ku,
Sendai 980-8578, Japan.
E-mail:
mtashiro@cyric.tohoku.ac.jp

The first two authors equally
contributed to this study.

ABSTRACT This study investigated the effects of the presence of a familiar pet dog on brain activity and psychophysiology in human volunteers. Fourteen participants (2 men, 12 women; mean age $\pm SD$ = 43.0 ± 10.8 years) were enrolled in the study. Uptake of ^{18}F-2-fluoro-2-deoxyglucose ([18F]FDG) on whole-brain positron emission tomography (PET) scans in the presence (but without interaction) and absence of their own pet dog was analyzed. In addition, an electrocardiograph was recorded to assess heart rate variability. Psychological condition was determined using the Stress Response Scale-18 (SRS-18). PET brain images were analyzed and compared between the two conditions (t-tests; $p < 0.001$) using a statistical parametric mapping program (SPM-5). Deactivated brain areas were detected in the left middle frontal gyrus (Brodmann area: BA 8), the right fusiform gyrus (BA 20), the left putamen, and the thalamus in the presence of the pet dog, indicating reduced regional brain activities associated with stress perception and sympathetic arousal. Similarly, SRS-18 scores were significantly lower ($p < 0.05$) in the presence of the pet dog, indicating a lowered stress response. However, autonomic function was not found to differ significantly between the two conditions. Overall, these results suggest that the participants were "relaxed" in the psychological sense. PET with [^{18}F]FDG appears to be a useful tool for examining the brain mechanisms underlying the psychophysiological well-being associated with the human–animal bond in terms of regional brain responses.

Anthrozoös   DOI: 10.2752/175303712X13240472427311

Keywords: autonomic function, brain activity, [18F]fluorodeoxyglucose ([18F]FDG), human–animal bond, positron emission tomography (PET)

 The partnership experienced between humans and animals, known as the human–animal bond, may have certain effects that relieve mental stress and anxiety in healthy as well as unhealthy individuals (Virues-Ortega and Buela-Casal 2006; O'Haire 2009). The relaxing effects of the human–animal bond have been studied in terms of autonomic nervous system functions. Vormbrock and Grossberg (1988) reported that the heart rate and blood pressure of human subjects decreased in the presence of a pet dog, which is suggestive of a relaxing effect. The human–animal bond may also have a substantial impact on basic emotions (moods and behaviors) in healthy individuals (Cole and Gawlinski 2000; Perkins et al. 2008). The relaxation and autonomic effects induced may be associated with central brain activity (Buchbauer et al. 1991; Alaoui-Ismaili et al. 1997). However, the neural mechanisms of the psychophysiological well-being in healthy participants in the presence of pet animals have not been studied in detail. The association of certain brain regions such as the anterior cingulated gyrus (ACG) and prefrontal cortex (PFC) with autonomic responses and emotion in general are suggested in the literature (Mak et al. 2009; Peelen, Atkinson and Vuilleumier 2010; Rahko et al. 2010). Therefore, it would be of interest to examine whether changes in regional brain activity relating to human emotion are induced in the presence of a pet animal.

Positron emission tomography (PET) with [18F]2-fluoro-2-deoxyglucose ([18F]FDG) is an established functional neuroimaging technique that can be used to determine regional brain activity in humans in vivo. [18F]FDG, a glucose analogue, is a tracer for measuring glucose metabolism, or cellular energy metabolism. By using PET with [18F]FDG (FDG PET), regional brain activity can be determined by the uptake of [18F]FDG during a period of about 30 to 40 min after intravenous administration (Masud et al. 2001; Duan et al. 2007; Tashiro et al. 2008). The highly sensitive 3D data acquisition mode of this imaging technique enables the psychophysiological status of humans to be assessed with minimal radiation exposure (lower than annual environmental exposure), and therefore is suitable for use in experimental studies involving human volunteers. Moreover, this method can show regional brain activity during rest and during specific task conditions (Masud et al. 2001; Duan et al. 2007). As such, it should be applicable to the comprehensive study of the effects on regional brain responses induced by the human–animal bond.

The presence of a pet animal may alter the autonomic nervous system functions related to relaxation. The autonomic changes that occur as a result of being in the presence of a pet can be determined by heart rate variability (HRV).

We hypothesized that the human–animal bond may alter central and autonomic nervous system activities and reduce psychological stress among pet owners. The aim of the present work was therefore to investigate the effects of the presence of a familiar pet dog on mood, autonomic nervous system functions and regional brain activity in healthy human volunteers. FDG PET was applied to evaluate the regional brain activity in static tasks: in the presence and absence of the participants' own pet dogs.

Methods
Participants
Fourteen healthy adults (2 men; 12 women; mean age ± *SD* = 43 ± 10.8 years, range 25–65 years), members of the Japanese Animal Hospital Association, were enrolled in this study.

These adults had indicated that they had no history of severe physical or psychiatric disorders. They were then examined by a medical doctor to ensure they did not have any of these problems. None of the candidates were excluded from the present study.

Written informed consent was obtained from all participants before starting the experiment. The night before the experiment, all participants were requested to take adequate rest and sleep, and to refrain from eating and drinking for at least 5 h prior to the start of the experiment. The study protocol was approved by the Ethics Committee of Tohoku University Graduate School of Medicine.

Study Design and PET Measurement

PET scans were conducted twice on one day with each participant (cross-over design). A 2-h interval separated the "task" condition (PET scan taken in the presence of their own pet dog) and the "resting control" condition (the PET scan taken while resting and in the absence of the dog), following the method validated previously by Nishizawa et al. (2001). The order of these conditions was counter-balanced across participants to minimize an "order effect," that is, a generalized effect on the study results associated with fixed ordering, such as participants feeling more intense anxiety during the first of the two PET scans, and a "carry-over" effect from the first to the second scan.

The participants were requested to sit comfortably on a chair with their eyes open at all times, in a dimly lit and quiet room. They were specifically instructed not to perform any kind of task during the 2-h interval (approximately) between the two scans and during the resting control condition without the dog present. In the task condition, participants were asked to sit, with their eyes open at all times, beside their dog without stroking or talking to him/her; however, compliance with these instructions was not fully monitored.

Two chest electrodes (Magnerode, TE-18: Fukuda Denshi Co., LTD., Tokyo, Japan) were attached to the participant's chest, over the manubrium sternum and apex (left 5th intercostal space, about 1 cm medial to the mid-clavicular line) for the evaluation of heart rate variability (HRV). A Teflon catheter was then inserted into the cubital vein of the right hand of each participant for intravenous administration of [^{18}F]FDG (mean 37.7 MBq for first scan and mean 74.5 MBq for second scan). Following the administration, the participants were instructed to sit quietly for 35 min on their own in the resting control condition or with their own dog in the task condition. To evaluate HRV, electrocardiograph (ECG) recordings were made using a polar 810i (Polar Electro Oy, Finland) for 30 min after the administration. Psychological status was measured using the self-report Stress Response Scale (SRS-18) before the PET scans were started (Suzuki et al. 1997). After 35 min of uptake of [^{18}F]FDG, all the electrodes were detached and the participants were requested to micturate before the PET scans were started.

For the PET scans, 40 min after the [^{18}F]FDG injection had been administered, the participants were asked to lie in the supine position on the PET scan table with their eyes open. The PET scan room was kept dimmed and quiet, and scanning was performed using a SET 2400 W PET scanner (Shimadzu, Kyoto, Japan) with an intrinsic spatial resolution of 3.9 mm full-width at half-maximum. The 3D whole-brain emission scan lasted for 15 min. The scan was taken from the orbitomeatal line to the vertex, depending on the participant's physique. A transmission scan (post-injection), which took 10 min to complete, was performed with a ^{68}Ge/^{68}Ga external rotating line source (370 MBq at purchase) to correct for the tissue attenuation of emitted photons. In total, PET scanning lasted for 25 min. The experimental design is summarized in Figure 1.

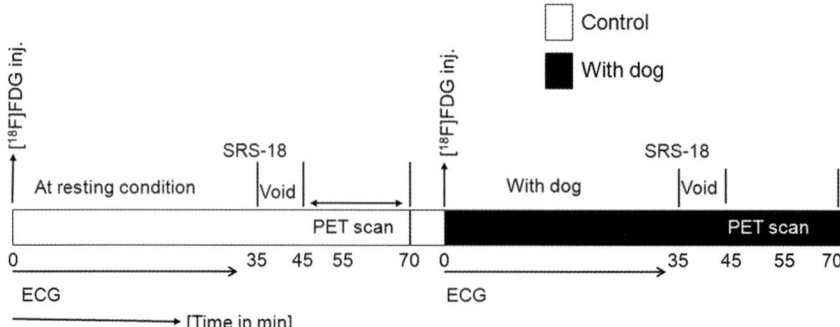

The order of the conditions was counter-balanced.

Figure 1. Schematic illustration of the study design.

Measurement of Psychological Stress

The SRS-18 was used to evaluate psychological stress between the task and resting control conditions. This 18-item scale, developed by Suzuki et al. (1997), measures psychological stress responses and consists of three subscales: "Depression/anxiety" (6 items), "Irritability/anger" (6 items), and "Helplessness" (6 items). Each item is evaluated on a 4-point scale (from 1 to 4), and for each subscale the score ranges from 6 to 24, with higher scores indicating higher levels of stress. For statistical examination, group comparisons of the SRS-18 scores between the control and task conditions were made using a non-parametric test (Wilcoxon Signed Rank Test), and the level of significance was set at $p < 0.05$.

Frequency-Domain Analysis of HRV

Frequency-domain analysis of HRV was conducted for evaluation of the sympathetic and parasympathetic nervous activities of the participants between the resting control and task conditions. HRV refers to the variation between two consecutive heartbeats, as assessed from RR intervals. Usually, the frequency of the peak R wave is taken to evaluate autonomic activity. The low frequency (LF: 0.04–0.15 Hz) and high frequency (HF: 0.15–0.4 Hz) spectral components of HRV are obtained for the evaluation of autonomic function (sympathetic and parasympathetic activity, respectively) (Task Force of the European Society of Cardiology and North American Society of Pacing and Electrophysiology 1996).

For analysis, we used HRV analytical software (University of Kuopio, Kuopio, Finland) (Niskanen et al. 2004). In this analytical procedure, a 30-min-long ECG record (control and task) was used. Consecutive heart beat intervals (R-R interval) of the ECG recordings were measured after determining the peak QRS complex, to obtain the LF and HF spectral components. HRV can be studied in the frequency domain by using a Fourier transformation to convert heart rate to the power spectrum (Niskanen et al. 2004). These LF and HF parameters were distinguished from frequency bands produced by power spectral analysis. The normalization values of LF (nLF) and HF (nHF) were used for the final elucidation of HRV data. The normalized LF (nLF) and HF (nHF) were determined according to the following formulas: nLF = LF / (LF + HF) and nHF = HF / (LF + HF), respectively (Robert 2007). Here, LF + HF is expressed as total power (TP).

PET Data Analysis

First, from each participant's brain image obtained in the second scan, the image from the first scan multiplied by a decay coefficient was subtracted. The decay coefficient was calculated based on the half-life of ^{18}F nuclide (110 min) and the length of the interval of 110 min (nearly 2 h) between the first and second scans (e.g., the decay coefficient was 0.5 when the interval was exactly 110 min).

The obtained pair of brain images for each participant was processed further using the statistical parametric mapping software package (SPM 5) (Friston et al. 1991, 1995). First, the PET images were spatially normalized to minimize the anatomical disparities between participants. An [^{18}F]FDG brain template from the Montreal Neurological Institute, McGill University, Canada (Friston et al. 1995) was used in this normalization procedure by applying affine and nonlinear transformations. Smoothing was performed with an [8, 8, 8] mm isotropic Gaussian filter kernel to compensate for errors in the spatial normalization. Voxel-based statistical analysis was performed on the smoothed images using a paired t-test, based on the general linear model, to detect the regional metabolic changes in brain activity between the task and resting control conditions. The threshold for significance was set at $p < 0.001$ without correction for multiple comparisons. The locations of relatively activated brain regions between the two conditions were identified with the standard x, y, and z coordinates (Talairach and Tournoux 1988).

Results

Participants' SRS-18 scores were significantly lower ($t = 2.07$, $p = 0.038$) in the task condition (with the dog) than in the resting control condition (Figure 2).

In the analysis of autonomic activities (sympathetic and parasympathetic: nLF and nHF) for the task and resting control conditions, nLF and nHF were found to be relatively stable ($t = 0.052$, $p = 0.958$; Figure 2), as evaluated by fast Fourier transform analysis.

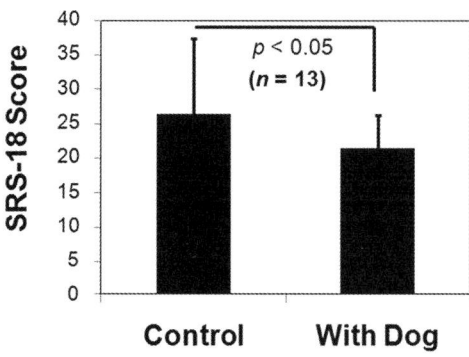

Figure 2. Psychological Stress Response Scale-18 scores of the participants while with and without (control) their dog. The higher the score, the higher the psychological stress.

Brain PET image data analysis revealed changes in regional brain activity between the task and resting control conditions ($p < 0.001$). Statistical parametric mapping results showed deactivated brain regions in the left middle frontal gyrus (Brodmann area 8: BA 8), right fusiform gyrus (BA 20), left putamen, and thalamus during the task condition compared with the resting control condition (Figure 4, Table 1); however, no activated brain areas were found in the task condition.

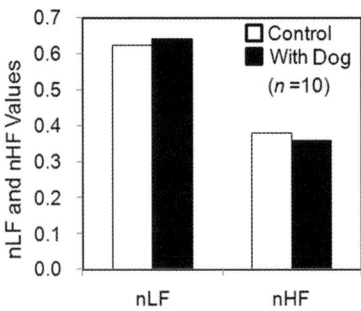

Figure 3. Heart rate variability (HRV) of participants while with (control) and without their dog, showing normalized units of low frequency and high frequency (nLF and nHF).

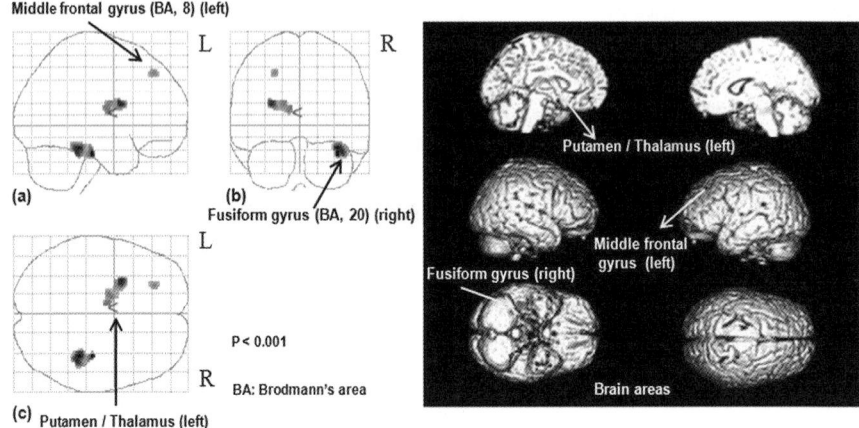

Figure 4. PET brain images showing areas where deactivation occurred when the participant was resting with their dog (statistical images produced based on 14 pairs of brain images): (a) the left middle frontal gyrus (Brodmman area 8: BA 8), (b) right fusiform gyrus (BA 20), and (c) subcortical structures (left putamen and thalamus) in the presence of the dog compared with its absence. Brain areas [middle frontal gyrus (left), fusiform gyrus (right), putamen/thalamus (left)] are shown in the volume rendering images (right images) (height threshold at $p < 0.001$, uncorrected for multiple comparisons; extent threshold of 10 voxel minimum).

Table 1. Regional brain deactivations with an accompanying animal (dog).

Regions	Broadmann's Area (BA)	Side	x, y, z (mm)	Z-value
Middle frontal gyrus	8	Left	−24, 38, 46	3.32
Fusiform gyrus	20	Right	36, −22, −24	4.31
Putamen		Left	−28, 6, 18	4.06
Thalamus		Left	−8, −8, 14	3.43

All areas were significant at $p < 0.001$.

Discussion

This is, to the best of the authors' knowledge, the first study that has attempted to elucidate the neurophysiology of the human–animal bond using PET imaging. In particular, the present investigation was conducted in order to evaluate the effects on mood, autonomic activity, and regional brain activity in humans when in the presence of a familiar pet. The significantly reduced SRS-18 scores suggest that the presence of a pet dog may improve the psychological state of the owner and relieve anxiety and stress, as discussed in previous studies (Vormbrock and Grossberg 1988; Raina et al. 1999; Cole and Gawlinski 2000; Virues-Ortega and Buela-Casal 2006; Perkins et al. 2008; O'Haire 2009). An interesting study by Raina et al (1999) also showed that individuals who own a pet animal have fewer health problems and considerably improved psychological well-being in the initial months of being a pet owner. Another study, related specifically to contact with a dog, postulates that the human–animal bond increases social behavior and decreases agitated behaviors (Perkins et al. 2008). Thus, the human–animal bond may have a substantial effect on psychophysiological status not only in healthy individuals but also in psychiatric patients. Barker and Dawson (1998) investigated the effects of the human–animal bond on 230 hospitalized psychiatric patients and compared the effect of a single 30-min-long animal companionship session. They found that the patients who had animal companionship showed significantly lower anxiety scores. Since no study had been conducted regarding the neural mechanism of the psychological improvement induced by the human–animal bond, the present functional neuroimaging study was conducted in healthy human volunteers as an exploratory study.

PET has been established as a suitable tool for assessing the psychophysiological status of healthy volunteers with minimal radiation exposure. Once the tracer for glucose metabolism [^{18}F]FDG has been administered, it is slowly transported to the brain tissue via glucose transporter proteins (GLUT) in around 30 to 40 min. In living cells, [^{18}F]FDG is metabolized into [^{18}F]FDG-6-phosphate in the presence of the enzymes hexokinase, or glucokinase. The [^{18}F]FDG-6-phosphate tends to accumulate in active tissues and thus reflects the degree of tissue glucose utilization. The pattern of the tissue glucose consumption is usually maintained for 1 or 2 h (metabolic trapping). Several PET studies have been conducted using this principle to demonstrate the difference between the resting condition and a static task such as aromatherapy (Duan et al. 2007; Masud et al. 2001) and a dynamic task such as a running exercise (Tashiro et al. 2008). From the results of the present study, FDG PET appears to be suitable for further understanding the effects of well-being induced by the human–animal bond in terms of the regional brain responses in healthy humans.

Voxel-by-voxel analysis of brain PET images in the present study revealed significantly deactivated brain regions in the left middle frontal gyrus (BA 8), right fusiform gyrus (BA 20), left putamen, and thalamus in the task condition compared with the resting control condition ($p < 0.001$), although we found no activated brain areas. This result can be explained by the observation in a previous study of decreased activity in the cerebral neocortex, such as in the frontal region, during a state of relaxation induced by aromatherapy (Duan et al. 2007). It is interesting to note that the frontal region also showed deactivation in the present study in spite of different laterality.

In addition, the lack of significant difference in the limbic regions might suggest that the stimulus intensity was not strong enough to show any difference between the two conditions.

This is supported, at least, by the fact that none of the brain regions directly related to autonomic tone (e.g., the anterior cingulate gyrus) were activated in the participants in the presence of their dog. In the above-mentioned study by Duan et al. (2007), in which participants received aromatherapy, several brain regions directly associated with the sense of smell were activated. In addition, Sinha et al. (2004) studied how emotional distress links with the central nervous system neural circuits in healthy human volunteers using fMRI. They found that specific striatal-limbic-prefrontal cortical circuits (caudate, putamen, thalamus, hippocampus, parahippocampal gyrus, and anterior and posterior cingulated gyrus) were involved in the regulation of emotional stress. Our study demonstrated deactivation of some of the structures of these striatal-limbic-prefrontal cortical circuits (putamen, thalamus and middle frontal gyrus), suggesting the reduction in emotional stress was induced by the presence of a familiar pet.

At this stage, however, there is still the possibility that the present deactivation patterns were non-specific ones obtained by type-I errors. Future replication is needed to draw a definitive conclusion and should serve to clarify the neural correlates of relaxation achieved by the human–animal bond.

On the other hand, the results of the participants' autonomic function, examined by the HRV method, showed no significant change in the parameters LF (low-frequency) and HF (high-frequency) between the two conditions, even though the previous study on relaxation effects due to aromatherapy did reveal significant HRV changes (Duan et al. 2007). The fact that nLF did not differ between the two conditions may suggest suppression of sympathetic tone (nLF), although it could also suggest that HRV measurement was not sensitive enough to detect this type of relaxation.

In addition to the problem of having used a relatively small sample size, there are other limitations. The present study design prevented the establishment of a uniform interpretation of the autonomic nervous activities induced by the presence of a pet dog. The interval between the first and second scan was short, and therefore the possibility of psychological "carry-over" effects cannot be ruled out completely, although we sought to minimize order effects. In addition, each participant was kept alone with his or her pet dog without any accompanying caregiver. Consequently, it is not known whether any situation occurred which might have prompted the participant to engage with their dog in physical activities, which could have potentially affected autonomic nervous system functions. It is known that HRV can be affected by participants' respiratory rate changes, but we did not measure this in this study. However, we believe that there would be few occasions in which irregular respiration would be induced while in the presence of the pet dog. This might be why autonomic nervous function was not seen to change much between the two conditions. Future studies should take these factors into account.

Future work should also address the issue of the "baseline" condition. Being in the *presence* of a familiar pet animal would be closer to the baseline state for most study participants living with pet animals than the "resting control" condition used in the present study, namely resting in the *absence* of the familiar pet animal. However, taking into account conventional research in the field of functional neuroimaging, this definition of the resting state (where participants remain alone) should be used as the "baseline" in future research, in order to avoid confusion. We believe, however, that the definition of the baseline condition may not ultimately affect the interpretation of the results obtained.

Conclusions

The present investigation evaluated the effects of the presence of a familiar pet dog on self-rated psychological stress and on autonomic activity and regional brain responses in humans. The results showed a significantly reduced psychological stress response and some deactivation in a few cerebral cortical and para-limbic regions in the presence of the pet. These results suggest that psychological well-being due to the presence of a pet animal may be associated with reduced activity in the cortical and para-limbic regions. The functional neuroimaging technique of PET appears to be a useful tool for examining the neural mechanisms underlying the human–animal bond.

Acknowledgements

This work was in part supported by Grants-in-Aid for scientific research (No. 21590754 for MT) from the Japan Society for the Promotion of Science (JSPS) in Japan, as well as by a grant from the Japan Society of Technology (JST) on research and education in "molecular imaging." We thank the Japanese Animal Hospital Association, Tokyo, Japan, for their support. Parts of the experimental results in this research were obtained using supercomputing resources at Cyberscience Center, Tohoku University. We also thank the volunteers for the PET study and Mrs Kazuko Takeda for taking care of the volunteers.

References

Alaoui-Ismaili, O., Varnet-Maury, E., Dittmar, A., Delhomme, G. and Chanel, J. 1997. Odor hedonics: Connection with emotional response estimated by autonomic parameters. *Chemical Senses* 22: 237–248.

Barker, S. B. and Dawson, K. S. 1998. The effects of animal-assisted therapy on anxiety ratings of hospitalized psychiatric patients. *Psychiatric Services* 49(6): 797–801.

Buchbauer, G., Jirovetz, L., Jager, W., Dietrich, H. and Plank, C. 1991. Aromatherapy: Evidence for sedative effects of the essential oil of lavender after inhalation. *Journal of Biosciences* 46: 1067–1072.

Cole, K. M. and Gawlinski, A. 2000. Animal-assisted therapy: The human–animal bond. *American Association of Critical Care Nurses Clinical Issues* 11(1): 139–149.

Duan, X., Tashiro, M., Wu, D., Yambe, T., Wang, Q., Sasaki, T., Kumagai, K., Luo, Y., Nitta, S. and Itoh, M. 2007. Autonomic nervous function and localization of cerebral activity during lavender aromatic immersion. *Technol Health Care* 15(2): 69–78.

Friston, K. J., Frith, C. D., Liddle, P. F. and Frackowiak, R. S. 1991. Comparing functional (PET) images: The assessment of significant change. *Journal of Cerebral Blood Flow & Metabolism* 11: 690–699.

Friston, K. J., Holmes, A. P., Worsley, K. J., Poline, J. P., Frith, C. D. and Frackowiak, R. S. 1995. Statistical parametric maps in functional imaging: A general linear approach. *Human Brain Mapping* 2: 189–210.

Mak, A. K., Hu, Z. G., Zhang, J. X., Xiao, Z. W. and Lee, T. M. 2009. Neural correlates of regulation of positive and negative emotions: An fmri study. *Neuroscience Letters* 457(2): 101–106.

Masud, M., Yamaguchi, K., Rikimaru, H., Tashiro, M., Ozaki, K., Watanuki, S., Miyake, M., Ido, T. and Itoh, M. 2001. Evaluation of resting brain conditions measured by two different methods (i.v. and oral administration) with F-18-FDG-PET. *Annals of Nuclear Medicine* 15(1): 69–73.

Nishizawa, S., Kuwabara, H., Ueno, M., Shimono, T., Toyoda, H. and Konishi, J. 2001. Double-injection FDG method to measure cerebral glucose metabolism twice in a single procedure. *Annals of Nuclear Medicine* 15(3): 203–207.

Niskanen, J. P. Tarvainen, M. P., Ranta-Aho, P. O. and Karjalainen, P. A. 2004. Software for advanced HRV analysis. *Computer Methods and Programs in Biomedicine* 76(1): 73–81.

O'Haire, M. 2009. The benefits of companion animals for human mental and physical health. RSPCA Australia Scientific Seminar, 1–9.

Peelen, M. V., Atkinson, A. P. and Vuilleumier, P. 2010. Supramodal representations of perceived emotions in the human brain. *Journal of Neuroscience* 30(30): 10127–10134.

Perkins, J., Bartlett, H., Travers, C. and Rand, J. 2008. Dog-assisted therapy for older people with dementia: A review. *Australasian Journal on Ageing* 27(4): 177–182.

Rahko, J., Paakki, J. J., Starck, T., Nikkinen, J., Remes, J., Hurtig, T., Kuusikko-Gauffin, S., Mattila, M. L., Jussila, K., Jansson-Verkasalo, E., Katsyri, J., Sams, M., Pauls, D., Ebeling, H., Moilanen, I., Tervonen, O. and Kiviniemi, V. 2010. Functional mapping of dynamic happy and fearful facial expression processing in adolescents. *Brain Imaging and Behavior* 4(2): 164–176.

Raina, P., Waltner-Toews, D., Bonnett, B., Woodward, C. and Abernathy, T. 1999. Influence of companion animals on the physical and psychological health of older people: An analysis of a one-year longitudinal study. *Journal of the American Geriatrics Society* 47(3): 323–329.

Robert, L. B. 2007. Interpretation of normalized spectral heart rate variability indices in sleep research: A critical review. *Sleep* 30(7): 913–919.

Sinha, R., Lacadie, C., Skudlarski, P. and Wexler, B. E. 2004. Neural circuits underlying emotional distress in humans. *Annals of the New York Academy of Sciences* 1032: 254–257.

Suzuki, S., Shimada, H., Miura, M., Katayanagi, K., Umano, R. and Sakano, Y. 1997. Development of a new psychological stress response scale (SRS-18) and investigation of the reliability and the validity. *Japanese Journal of Behavioral Medicine* 4: 22–29.

Talairach, J. and Tournoux, P. 1988. *Co-planner Stereotaxic Atlas of the Human Brain.* M. Rayport (translator), Stuttgart: Thieme.

Tashiro, M., Itoh, M., Fujimoto, T., Masud, M. M., Watanuki, S. and Yanai, K. 2008. Application of positron emission tomography to neuroimaging in sports sciences. *Methods* 45(4): 300–306.

Task Force of the European Society of Cardiology and North American Society of Pacing and Electrophysiology. 1996. Heart rate variability—standards of measurement, physiological interception, and clinical use. *Circulation* 93(5): 1043–1065.

Virues-Ortega, J. and Buela-Casal, G. 2006. Psychophysiological effects of human–animal interaction: Theoretical issues and long-term interaction effects. *Journal of Nervous and Mental Diseases* 194(1): 52–57.

Vormbrock, J. K. and Grossberg, J. M. 1988. Cardiovascular effects of human–pet dog interactions. *Journal of Behavioral Medicine* 11(5): 509–517.

ANTHROZOÖS
VOLUME 25, ISSUE 1
PP. 35–48

REPRINTS AVAILABLE
DIRECTLY FROM
THE PUBLISHERS

PHOTOCOPYING
PERMITTED
BY LICENSE ONLY

Owning the Problem: Media Portrayals of Overweight Dogs and the Shared Determinants of the Health of Human and Companion Animal Populations

Chris Degeling and Melanie Rock

Population Health Intervention Research Centre, University of Calgary, Calgary, Canada

*Address for correspondence:
Dr Chris Degeling,
Population Health Intervention Research Centre,
University of Calgary,
Teaching, Research and
Wellness Building Room
3E15, 3280 Hospital Drive
NW, Calgary, AB, Canada
T2N 4Z6.
E-mail: cjdegeli@ucalgary.ca*

ABSTRACT Weight-related health problems have become a common topic in Western mass media. News coverage has also extended to overweight pets, particularly since 2003 when the US National Academy of Sciences announced that obesity was also afflicting co-habiting companion animals in record numbers. To characterize and track views in popular circulation on causes, consequences, and responsibilities vis-à-vis weight gain and obesity, in pets as well as in people, this study examines portrayals of overweight dogs that appeared from 2000 through 2009 in British, American, and Australian mass media. The ethnographic content analysis drew inspiration from the literature in population health, animal–human relationships, communication framing, and the active nature of texts in cosmopolitan societies. Three main types of media articles about overweight dogs appeared during this period: 1) reports emphasizing facts and figures; 2) stories emphasizing personal prescriptions for dog owners, and 3) societal critiques. To help ordinary people make sense of canine obesity, media articles often highlight that dogs share the lifestyle of their human companion or owner, yet the implications of shared social and physical environments is rarely considered when it comes to solutions. Instead, media coverage exhorts people who share their lives with overweight dogs to "own the problem" and, with resolve, to normalize their dog's physical condition by imposing dietary, exercise, and relationship changes, thereby individualizing culpability rather than linking it to broader systemic issues.

Keywords: companion animals, media, narrative analysis, obesity, public understanding

Anthrozoös DOI: 10.2752/175303712X13240472427230

In 2001, the US Surgeon General issued an urgent "Call for Action" to quell what he termed an emerging epidemic of obesity (US Department of Health and Human Services 2001). This report not only incited a rapid escalation in research on human obesity, but also galvanized public, political, and media interest in the issue (Kersh and Morone 2005; Oliver and Lee 2005). And yet recent expressions of concern among researchers and in the media about the health effects of excess weight have not been confined to human populations, but also the increasing incidence of obesity amongst our co-habiting companion animals. In 2003, a committee of the US National Academy of Sciences reported that one in four dogs and cats worldwide were overweight (National Research Council 2003), which helped to lend a pet angle to global media coverage of weight gain and obesity. Armed with this report and related findings (McGreevy et al. 2005; Lund et al. 2006), veterinary opinion leaders and animal welfare advocates have managed to harness media interest in obesity—in concert with their enduring fascination with matters animal—thus raising the public profile of an emerging pet health issue. This paper addresses the mass media's role in connecting weight gain in dogs with human activity and social organization. Following on from studies of the influence of comparative metaphors and analogies on lay-people's perceptions of human obesity (Barry et al. 2009), it is likely that media portrayals of overweight pets have the potential to have an effect on the general public's understanding of, and engagement with, the determinants of health—in canine as well as in human populations.

Pets and People—Shared Lives, Shared Environments, Shared Health Concerns

Pet animals occupy an important place in many Western societies (Franklin 1999). Almost 50% of households in North America, Europe and Australasia include one or more animal companions. Almost half of these animals—and their owners—will see a veterinarian at least annually. These interactions between humans, animals, and health care providers have effects that extend beyond the well-being of individual pets. People's ways of thinking about pet health cannot be understood without reference to how they think about human health—their own health but also the health of others (family, friends, and entire populations). When it comes to pets, people compare and contrast. Partly they are actively encouraged to do so, for example in veterinary clinics. But more generally people make comparisons because they regard their pets as beings that resemble humans—physically as well as emotionally or spiritually. People will often go to extraordinary lengths to care for a pet, for example, by seeking specialist veterinary services and by rearranging their schedules to follow through on veterinary advice to administer medication twice or more per day. While not all pet owners are prepared or equipped financially to provide the highest standards of veterinary healthcare, expectations regarding pet health are shifting—not least for recognized health risks such as over-feeding and obesity.

Previous studies of human–canine interactions vis-à-vis weight gain and obesity have sought to establish whether overweight people tend to have overweight dogs, to predict which people over-feed their dogs, and to identify enablers and barriers to regular dog-walking (Cutt et al. 2007; Nijland, Stam and Seidell 2010; Rohlf et al. 2010). Our approach differs, in that we look to media coverage as a site that amplifies particular ways of thinking about why so many people and dogs in Western societies are overweight, and what can or should be done in response. There is an extensive literature on obesity and health in human populations where the demonstrated root-causes now include genetic factors, diet, levels of physical activity, and how an individual's behavior on these dimensions is mediated by their social and economic circumstances (McLaren 2007; James 2008). Against this background our central premise is that the rising incidence of weight-related health problems in co-habiting human and canine populations are related, due to socio-cultural and economic forces that structure people's everyday lives and that influence how people exercise agency, including how people regard and interact with dogs.

Health News, Animal–Human Interest Stories and Active Texts

Media content can reflect prominent social concerns and changes in the nature and tone of popular discourses. As well as showing that "something is happening" in a society, news reports can have recursive effects. For example, numerous studies indicate that the media plays a prominent role in how the public understand issues relating to health (Brodie et al. 2003; Wang and Gantz 2007). In essence, media reports are forms of communication that inform people's knowledge and perceptions, and thereby can also inform their actions and reactions. As an issue emerges and then becomes widely viewed as a significant health problem, individuals rely on media depictions, political filters, and personal experiences to gather and synthesize information (Entman and Herbst 2001). Explanations provided by professionals and institutions tend to be prominent in media coverage of health issues, and may be cited authoritatively or criticized. For example, media coverage of the emergence of Methicillin-resistant Staphylococcus-aureus (MRSA) has acted as a "bridge" between medical findings and public perceptions, entrenching the notion that mismanagement of the UK's National Health Service has contributed to the problem of this "hospital superbug" (Washer and Joffe 2006). Notably— as with many recently emerged and important health issues (Blue and Rock 2011)—the MRSA situation and media profile in the UK also has a pet angle. Aside from expressions of concern about over-prescription of antibiotics by veterinarians, there were also news-reports that individualized the story around the fate of a prominent companion animal. When a dog named "Bella" contracted MRSA and died shortly after undergoing surgery in 2004, her actress owner also blamed organizational routines and hospital mismanagement in the veterinary context, for giving her animal this infection (Gardiner 2009). This situation led to the creation of a not-for-profit foundation whose activities include hosting a popular website that provides information about MRSA in pets as well as in people, including reposts of media coverage on the topic.

Conceptually and methodologically, this paper builds on previous work on animal–human interest stories in cosmopolitan societies (Podberscek 1994; Franklin and White 2001). Like reports of new cancer risks or medical breakthroughs, variations of "man-bites-dog" stories are a news staple (Hughes 1940). Uncanny, endearing or horrifying tales about pets appear in the media almost every day. We posit that popular interest in dogs and obesity combine in media coverage, and that such news-reporting conveys information and perspectives that ordinary people readily apply to themselves, to their friends and families, and to human populations more generally. Following on from Foucault as well as from Gramsci, the study of texts can provide insights into how activity at one place and time relate to what has occurred and continues to occur elsewhere (Smith 1999; Mykhalovskiy 2003). We thus regard our media corpus as the result of—and impetus for—sets of social practices. This way of conceiving of texts is less concerned with manifest content and more concerned with how particular texts originate from, represent, and help to shape everyday life through their powers of persuasion, and/or by inciting disagreement and the production of further texts and other activities and discourses.

Regarding the co-incidence throughout the Western world of health problems linked to being overweight in human and canine populations, our concern with active texts and with animal–human interest stories more specifically is germane because people *do* a great deal with, for, and on behalf of these animals. They buy toothbrushes for their dogs, sleep with them, carry around photos of them in their wallets, criticize the behavior of other people's dogs, and donate money, time, or both to animal welfare organizations. The everyday ways in which people go about caring for animals means that pet care is a key way in which people may come to understand and to engage with health science. From this vantage point, whether and how newspapers report on fat dogs and on fatness among dogs may matter a great deal. And yet it is difficult to measure and describe how media reports effect the practices of the reading public. With this caveat in mind, our aim is twofold. First, we investigate how the causes, consequences, meanings, and solutions to weight-related issues in pet animal populations are construed in media coverage, and then we consider how this reporting connects with issues pertaining to human affairs and human health.

Methods
Data Sources and Collection
A search of EBSCOhost Newspaper Source (US) for articles published between 2000 and 2009 containing the terms "dog*," "canine*," or "pet*" and "overweight," "obese*," or "fat" was undertaken, which led to identifying a total of 213 unique articles about overweight dogs. This database covers a wide selection of national and regional newspapers in Britain, Australia, and North America, as well as transcripts from several US broadcasters, including CBS News, FOX News, and NPR. The 213 articles were downloaded as full-text and then manually catalogued as to their year and national origin.

Data Analysis
This study is based on ethnographic content analysis (ECA). With this method, researchers seek to interpret text and images within the context of their use (Altheide 1987; Krippendorff 2004). Drawing on both numerical and narrative data, the aim is to provide rich descriptions and comparisons of the ways in which specific forms of communication provide causal interpretations, promote particular viewpoints and moral evaluations, and provide prescriptive solutions. ECA is particularly useful as a means to elucidate patterns in how issues are "anchored" and "framed." Any attempt to describe and explain a new phenomenon such as an emerging burden of disease must rely upon analogies, comparisons and metaphors. Reporters often seek to "anchor" emerging issues in terms and concepts that are familiar to the reader to make them easier to understand—the media coverage of SARS frequently comparing the epidemic to the Spanish Influenza of 1918 is a pertinent example (Moscovici 2000; Washer 2004). Once anchored in familiar terms and events, different types of information and perspectives are emphasized at the expense of others. Some elements are "framed in" while others are "framed out." In essence, communicative frames a) define problems, b) diagnose causes, c) provide some normative assessment of the situation, and d) suggest solutions and remedies (Entman 1993, p. 52). In combination, these comparisons and pieces of salient information serve to provide meaning, tell us what to do, and provide an account of who is at risk, who is "other," and, ultimately, who is to blame. A given communicative utterance or text may not contain all four elements, or not explicitly, but even a rather small corpus on a particular topic is likely to exhibit framing patterns and these frames are likely to have been "borrowed."

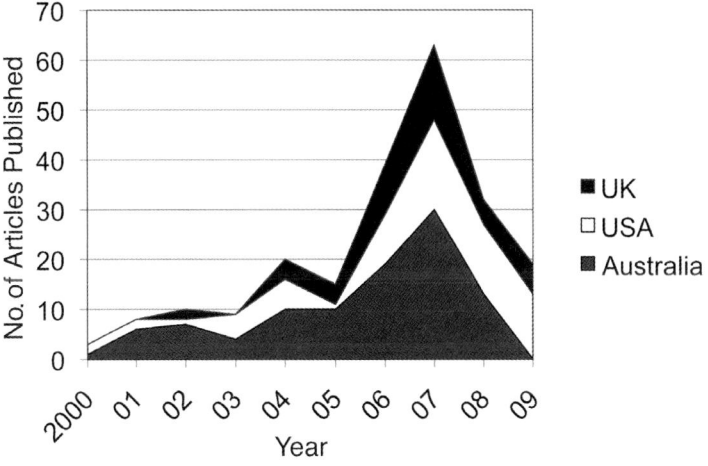

Figure 1. A "stacked" table of year by year and national differences in the number of articles addressing the issue of canine obesity published in our corpus of newspapers from the UK, Australia, and the USA (2000–2009).

With these concepts and textual relationships in mind, our analysis of the 213 articles on overweight dogs proceeded through several cycles of immersion and crystallization of insights—a research process comprised of repeated readings and comparisons across and between news-markets, discussions amongst the authors, periods of testing of alternate explanations, and then re-immersion within the research materials (Borkan 1999; LeCompte and Schensul 1999).

Results

Media interest in overweight dogs had emerged by 2002, had built momentum by 2004, peaked in 2007, and had tapered off by 2009 (see Figure 1). The peak in 2007 can be attributed to a constellation of events that attracted interest across the news-markets examined. These include: the release of diet pills for dogs; a series of high-profile animal welfare prosecutions involving obese animals; and a number of global recalls of popular brands of pet foods. Differences in magnitude across the three marketplaces are evident, with the most interest shown in Australia (which tended to report on events in the other markets), followed by the more inward-looking US, and then by the UK.

It is notable that most of the news reporting we examined used puns in the headlines and news-banners. This is fairly typical of animal stories and most other human-interest pieces in newspapers. However, very rarely was the jocular tone carried into the body of the article. Instead our analysis distilled three patterns in how the media has chosen to use the animal-interest genre to frame the complex issues surrounding the increasing prominence of canine obesity. Media reports tended to focus upon one of the following: facts and figures, personal prescriptions, and societal critiques. It is important to emphasize that these tropes did not necessarily occur in sequence or remain entirely distinct. As early as 2004, for example, societal critiques occasionally appear in direct response to the facts and figures. Yet over time, the meaning of an increasing incidence of overweight dogs developed into a recognizable discourse, one that emphasized individual responsibility.

Look! Another Obesity Epidemic

The first type of story to appear centered on "facts and figures" and were typically sparked by a statistical study or survey. A university researcher, scientific institution, pet health insurance company, or animal welfare charity had circulated a media release to publicize their findings, and access to one of the researchers or a prominent member of the organization was also provided as an expert interview subject. For example, the following report appeared in *The Sunday Telegraph*, the largest-circulation weekend paper in Sydney, Australia:

> A BALLOONING obesity rate among Australians is spreading to our four-footed friends, latest figures show. More than 40 per cent of dogs and 20 per cent of cats are overweight or obese, the RSPCA says. Animal experts claim Australia's inactive lifestyle and poor diet is killing our furry friends. They are dying of heart disease, diabetes and arthritis—the same weight-related disorders as humans … The RSPCA recommends walking dogs for around 30 minutes each day and following a healthy diet. (Sexton 2004, p. L34)

The same "facts and figures" type of story appeared in British and US media, heralding the existence of a "second wave" obesity epidemic occurring in pet populations: "The best solution to overweight pets and overweight pet owners is the same: Eat less and exercise more" ("Our doggies, ourselves" 2006, p. D10). The apparent co-incidence of a human obesity is mentioned prominently to provide context and to anchor the story for readers. These articles consistently feature a "why should we care" component, which highlights health risks for overweight pets as a prelude to underscoring a need for self-reflection followed by immediate action on the part of animal owners. What seems to unify the recommendations offered in "facts and figures" reports is the underlying supposition that dog owners were unaware of the problem and the risks it posed, so that correcting deficiencies in knowledge would be enough to spur them to "ensure daily exercise, limit food intake." This type of recommendation was often followed by a pointed observation related to the owner's health, such as "they could do worse than apply the same regimen to themselves" (Hamilton 2004, p. 9).

Pets Pay the Price for Individuals' Failings

Whereas "facts and figures" articles tended to be brief, to center on statistical findings, and to end with exhortations for dog owners, the second variety of media articles in our corpus emphasize "personal prescriptions." These accounts of canine obesity step inside the facts and figures to look in greater depth at causes and solutions. This type of article typically cites both veterinarians and owners. Articles typically begin by citing owners, who attest to their previous ignorance, guilt, or frustration at the weight and overall state of their dog. Veterinarians—either a local practitioner or one who works for a university or animal welfare organization—then recount their experiences of the canine obesity epidemic and reiterate the nature of the risks posed by excessive weight for canine health. In addition, veterinary sources often give their opinion of the behavior and choices of an archetypical owner of an overweight animal. The co-incidence of human and animal obesity in the same household is often used to make a number of different types of claims, such as: "overweight people inflict their poor lifestyle on their pets" (Bee 2005, p. 8). Alternatively, there are occasionally statements from experts in line with what Bourdieu (1995) described as a "shared way of being" or *habitus*, but without reference to hierarchy in human populations, such as this observation in *USA Today*:

Many pets lounge around the house all day and then join other members of the family for snacks in front of the tube at night. (Fackelmann 2003, p. L9)

A series of contributing factors are usually mentioned, which often included: the calorie-rich nature of modern pet foods; an escalation in "treat culture," (Miller 1998, pp. 40–49) that is, the tendency for each shopping trip to include the purchase of small extravagances directed toward a particular member of the household (dogs, in this case); longer periods of time spent away from the home for paid employment; and passive pastimes among dog owners, such as the television example given above. Only very occasionally are demographic changes (e.g., single-person households) and urbanization (e.g., confined apartment living) mentioned as being contributors to the increasing numbers of overweight dogs. Notably, attempts to tie the causal elements described above together were rare in our corpus. The stories are anchored by comparisons between the every-day routines of individual pets and the presumed consequences of owner lifestyles.

Within these prescriptive articles, the narrative tends to shift between tales of unhealthy love and unthinking neglect or cruelty. The cause of excess weight in pet animals is then individualized—using some or all of these normative elements—as a deficit of the owner in two slightly different ways. Either owners are presumed to be deficient in their knowledge about diet, physical activity, and what constitutes a healthy body condition for a dog; or they are presumed to be deficient in the type of relationship that they have allowed to form with their dog. In both instances, the problem is construed as a moral failing that requires behavioral discipline and control on the part of individual owners. This focus on owner control and responsibility, or the lack of it, is usually given a veterinary imprimatur. For example, a veterinarian interviewed by the *Charleston Gazette* (US) of West Virginia was at pains to point out who was the responsible party:

[W]e control the situation ... Dogs and cats can't open the refrigerator. They can't have a midnight snack unless you provide it. (Morgan 2006)

Overweight dogs are sometimes granted considerable agency in this dynamic, to the point of being described as manipulative, demanding, and even glutinous individuals, particularly in the Australian media. For one *Herald Sun* (Australia) reporter, as an example, devious pets were even deliberately: "emotionally blackmailing their gullible owners for an extra snack and are becoming obese in the process" (Trumble 2006, p. 35). These types of stories also serve to account for the intransigence of canine obesity to scientifically designed diet dog food. The result is that rather than a lack of knowledge, the central problem is now construed as owner psychology. Overarching these assessments of owner conduct, the message is—in short—that some people are so ill-disciplined that they are giving "human" diseases to their dogs. Once blame has been assigned to individual owners, the "prescription" is to modify the animals eating, exercise it regularly, and take steps to redress any pathological power-relations in human–dog interactions. The key message is that these animals are paying for the failings of individuals: their ignorance, weakness, laziness, overindulgence, or combinations thereof.

Pills for Podgy Pets—All a Step Too Far

The third and final variety of story in our corpus explores the implications of a canine obesity epidemic for the Western way of life. These articles comprise either satirical communiqués or general commentaries. The causal account offered is not about individuals but society as a whole, yet with little or no reference to social inequality. The problem is construed as pathological over-consumption. Consequently, these articles use the story of companion animal obesity as an anchor or exemplar in order to make broader comments on scientific, legislative, or business reactions to the pet animal weight "crisis." Yet in the end, the preferred solution is individual behavioral change. An editorial in the *New York Times* exemplifies this evolving trope:

> It's obviously time for a war on pet gluttony. Perhaps a nation that stashes its prized pets in canine day-care centers, sends them to doggie psychiatrists, and buries them in special cemeteries will rise to the challenge by establishing health clubs for pets with special trainers. Alternatively, the human couch potatoes who contribute to this problem could put down the report, get the leash, and take Fido for a run. ("Porky pets" 2003, p. 18)

Normative assessments can then be made about the part being played by one or more institutions in escalating or responding to the situation. As an illustration, by the end of 2005 a features writer at *The Times* (UK) professed to be tiring of the "spin-cycle" following the release of yet another survey and press release from an animal healthcare provider, in this case the Chartered Society of Physiotherapists (CSP). In Alan Coren's Christmas message, he notes:

> Eighty-one percent of canine Britons, declared the CSP this week, are obese … This survey has me worried, as surveys invariably do. That is what surveys are for … Hang on I hear 23 per cent of my readership fretfully cry, what about our beloved moggies. Oh do leave off: you of all pet lovers know that cats are canny, circumspect self-preservationists … Unless, of course, they happen to live with an animal dumb enough to put up a big wobbly tree and hang bright dangly balls all over it. (Coren 2005, p. 17)

Aside from the examples of consumerist exasperation and survey fatigue provided above, discourse surrounding the issue of companion animal obesity has also been used as an anchor from which to target: the intrusive role of state legislation (Derbyshire 2008); and the anthropomorphism and sentimentality of modern human–pet relationships (Harper 2007). The apparent aim of anchoring these opinion pieces on overweight dogs is to raise the question: is more than companion animal health at risk from these developments? Although the column or opinion piece rarely provides an answer to this existential enquiry, they rarely resist positing a need to return to commonsense solutions. As much as these articles tend to point to a systemic context for canine obesity, blame is still individualized. Any gesture towards distal over proximal causation was framed as a "step too far."

As the decade progressed, the issue of canine obesity became intertwined and began to reciprocally shape the concerns of veterinarians, the pet food industry, animal welfare organizations, and pharmaceutical companies. By end of the decade, the terse expression "sedentary lifestyles" often substitutes for any discussion of the shared social and structural determinants of obesity, and implicitly becomes a short-hand code for the "busyness" and "laziness" of contemporary dog-owning populations. It is notable that during the period under study, the issues and agendas that activated media coverage of canine obesity differed somewhat by country. For example, the US media placed far more importance than the UK or Australian coverage on nutrition and commercial pet-food. This media focus was already present when, in early 2007, a global recall of Hills© products heightened concerns about the regulation and ingredient sources of the pet food industry. Although the Hills© recall was never linked directly with canine obesity, it would seem that news coverage surrounding tainted pet food began to influence the content and tone of stories about canine obesity in US news-reports. Furthermore, caring for an overweight dog sometimes occasioned discussion of human diets and the food industry. A Ms Newell summed up the nub of this issue for the *Dallas Morning News*: "I don't have perfect eating habits, either ... How am I supposed to expect my dog to?" (Menzer 2007).

Whereas the media in the US and UK tend to focus on local developments, the results of British surveys, legislative amendments, and animal welfare cases—as well as American Insurance Company reports and pharmaceutical innovations—invariably elicited a response from the Australian media. Nevertheless, these developments are only ever used to provide context, because, in the words of Dr Hugh Wirth, the problem of pet obesity in Australia "begins and ends with the owner" (Skotnicki 2004, p. 32). Consequently, the focus remains on describing and evaluating human–animal interactions and, ultimately, animal owners. In contrast, in the UK, the story of the unfolding canine epidemic becomes coupled with coverage of the legal and legislative activities and agendas of its main animal welfare organization, the Royal Society for the Prevention of Cruelty to Animals, or RSPCA. Notable events included high-profile prosecutions of owners who had failed to take steps to manage the weight of their morbidly-obese pets. In the UK, canine obesity came to be framed explicitly as an issue of animal welfare. Indeed, "fat dogs" become the central focus in media depictions of amendments to the British Animal Welfare Act (Derbyshire 2008). The British newspapers leave little unexplored, reporting on everything from the high levels of anxiety amongst the owners of overweight animal who fear punitive action to anger amongst dog lovers who are incensed at the number of animals sacrificed during development, testing, and registration of any possible pharmaceutical solutions.

In addition to the Hills© recall of 2007, another important development in the same year contributed directly to media coverage of overweight dogs. In January 2007, the multinational pharmaceutical company Pfizer© announced FDA approval for Slentrol®, a weight-loss medication for dogs. The drug—an appetite suppressant—was explicitly marketed as being a useful tool for veterinarians and animal owners to gain control of a dog's weight when diet modification and increased exercise could not be implemented successfully. In many ways a publicist's dream, the news of a "diet pill for dogs" attracted worldwide attention. Notably, the Australian media coverage of the new drug remained focused on the human–animal relationship, and the responsibility and relative agency of owners to make the right choices for their pets. In one instance, the drug was described in an Australian paper as "a cop-out for dog owners" who were too lazy to commit to feeding and exercising their dog more appropriately (Lallo 2007). By comparison, in the US, despite the personal endorsement of the head of the animal division of the FDA, news of the drug activated further reflection upon the state of American society. As other papers described the ready-made market and potential uses of the canine medication, an editor at South Dakota's *Aberdeen American News* opined:

> The development of diet pills for dogs should be a real eye opener to all of us.
> Our society has become increasingly reliant on quick fixes for everything ... It is
> time for Americans to start retaking control of their lives. ("Dogs don't need diet
> pills, need disciplined care" 2007)

In the UK, meanwhile, the introduction of a weight-loss drug for dogs was framed by an existing discourse on owner neglect. In fact, the RSPCA—largely responsible for generating the data that established the existence of a canine obesity epidemic—opposed the use of a canine weight-loss drug, so as to prevent it from being used to disguise more pressing animal welfare issues. What these differences in the coverage of Slentrol® indicate is that in the UK, canine obesity is most likely to be considered a moral and personal failing of the owner, requiring the existence of punitive animal welfare legislation for extreme cases and to serve as a deterrent. In Australia, the condition is indicative of an owner who needs further education to establish appropriate relationships around food and to encourage healthy human–pet interactions. In the US—where the drug received a less hostile reaction from veterinary professionals— owning a fat dog was construed in media sources as indicative of a loss of control which requires careful consideration of consumption patterns. As the advocates, critics, and cynics described above invariably pointed out, with a pharmaceutical intervention, the appearance of normalcy can, if necessary, be restored but without rooting out the pathogenesis.

Discussion

Historical studies indicate that concerns about animal welfare mirror or even foreshadow broader social concerns (Turner 1980). In other words, studying the history of animal welfare has proved to be a way of studying deeply rooted values, structures, and tensions (Tester 1991). In this paper we adopt a similar approach to overweight dogs. More precisely we have analyzed the problematization of fatness through the lens of newspaper accounts of canine obesity. The main reason why we think that these media portrayals are of consequence is that we view such texts as socially active. In other words, newspaper stories not only reflect particular ways of thinking, they also imply particular ways of understanding and reacting—in the act of reading, but also in other spheres of activity. In much the same way prominent scientific and media discourses around obesity have been shown to be shaping how Canadian youth conceive of the relationship between people's body-type and their health status (Rail, Holmes and Murray 2010), the news-stories in our corpus on canine weight might induce some people to speculate on the psychological fitness and exercise habits of others, thus influencing social interactions.

Weight gain and obesity in human populations consistently "anchored" the media coverage in our corpus, yet differences and frank social inequalities in the distribution of weight status were invariably "framed out" while individual behavior was "framed in" as the preferred solution and a moral obligation. Even when societal causes received acknowledgement, moral responsibility remained firmly vested in individuals. Medicalizing problems can sometimes absolve people of blame for sickness, but not in this case. Only those capable of resisting powerful societal forces seem to be appropriate candidates for dog ownership, according to these media portrayals, at a time when a growing body of evidence suggests that dogs can promote health in urbanized populations. While some articles mentioned causal factors such as urban design and television-viewing, none emphasized policy reforms or community development as solutions. Even in the handful of news-reports in the sample promoting the health benefits of walking the dog, the prescription was that individuals must own their pets—and thereby their own—weight-related problems. Yet plausible interventions that could promote canine as well as human health include: dog-walking clubs (to help owners to build social networks and to enable non-owners to share in the health benefits of dog-walking), telecommuting (to encourage people to walk a dog during off-peak hours of the day, which could also help to reduce traffic congestion and air pollution), improved lighting in streets and parks (to make it easier for people to walk a dog in the evening), preferred zoning near workplaces for dog daycare programs (to allow people to walk a dog over lunch, for example), and allowing dogs on public transit (so that dogs and their owners could walk at least part of the way to workplaces).

Ethnographic content analysis is explicitly and reflexively attuned to accounting for social relations that help to shape texts as well as their influence in practice (Altheide 1987). This emphasis on social relations and practices is important because media coverage does not exist in isolation but instead is actively and iteratively interpreted in light of other trends, news, and events. For our purposes, the most important corollary is the rising incidence of weight-related health problems in human populations. While we have discerned patterns in source types and main messages in our corpus, we have not attempted to isolate or quantify these differences in any precise way. Our intent has been to examine notions in popular circulation about health from a novel angle—overweight dogs—not to measure their frequency. In any case, we found that the media accounts consistently individualized responsibility for weight-related health problems in both dogs and people.

Human–Animal Comparisons

Media research on recent infectious epidemics provides a number of interesting comparisons, especially as these stories often have a prominent animal angle. Examinations of the response of British newspapers to new diseases such as SARS and MRSA points to frames in which the risk of catching these conditions is externalized by linking disease origins and blame to "others." While the threat of SARS soon became something that "filthy" Chinese householders face, Peter Washer finds that aside from descriptions of superbugs as "nature's revenge" for the modern way of living, media reports about MRSA eventually tend not to focus on the origin of the condition, but upon the management practices of the British healthcare system deemed to be responsible for its spread (Washer 2004; Washer and Joffe 2006). A similar trope emerges in Washer's (2006) subsequent examination of representations of mad cow disease in British newspapers. Similar to canine obesity, in UK media coverage of BSE and MRSA, there is not an immediate or obvious external "other" to blame. Pointedly, in media coverage of non-infectious epidemic amongst a co-habiting pet animal population, the "others" held responsible are individual owners. The spread of the condition is portrayed as a socially mediated process that afflicts dogs owned by problematic types of people. This species jump means that we have veterinary epidemiological data being used in animal-interest stories to support causal claims and normative assertions as to obesogenic attributes of the values, living standards, and choices of certain segments of the human population. In these terms, the only difference between obesity in owners and their companion animals is the presumed ability of humans to restrain themselves, and exercise choice on the behalf of dependent others.

Precisely because dogs occupy a different social position than that of a rational, informed, and autonomous consumer, it is striking how closely our findings resemble results from survey-based research on public perceptions of overweight and obese children. Investigations of public perceptions in Australia (Covic, Roufeil and Dziurawiec 2007) and in North America (Evans et al. 2005; Potestio et al. 2008) indicate that most citizens understand obesity to have complex causes. Even so, they place more importance on the parents, food, and sedentary pastimes in determining the incidence of overweight children than on structural or systemic factors. Thus, their preferred remedy is parental action. Similarly, media and professional discourses of neglect and moral failure are currently evolving in the UK in relation to the parents of overweight children (Viner et al. 2010). And yet the individualization of culpability is at odds with current thinking amongst the scientific and public health community about root causes (Foresight Report 2007; Maziak, Ward and Stockton 2008). As the medical sociologist Regina

Lawrence (2004) identifies, the overarching distinction between "behavioral" and "environmental" stories about obesity is that they either "individualize" blame, or contextualize excessive body weight as a "systemic" problem. Whether the focus is on individuals or their context has important implications for any normative assessments, public opinions about policy prescriptions, and attempts at intervention (Saguy and Almeling 2008).

Conclusions

How issues are framed in public discussions matters. Media reports are not a simple neutral account but are socially active. A newspaper story might induce someone to take the time and effort to prepare their own pet food, speculate on the diet and exercise habits of others, or volunteer for an animal welfare charity, and influence in what capacity. What we see in the media coverage of canine obesity is the use of the animal-interest stories to communicate ideas about consumption, care, responsibility, and their relationship to excess weight in urban "sedentary" populations. It is notable that while systemic factors and environmental contexts are considered to be causal contributors, the owner's (in)ability to change a lack of time and/or space to exercise; animal by-laws; and perceptions of neighborhood safety are uniformly downplayed in the media. When it comes to the causes and consequences of canine obesity, the main message is that individual owners need to own the problem. The proof of the owner's control and success is in the pudding, so to speak, of their dog's weight. These types of prescriptive assertions lead to the most surprising finding of our study. Media depictions commonly use connections and correlations in environmental context between people and pets to anchor stories on canine obesity, but the possible implications of this shared health risk remain almost entirely unexamined when it comes to solutions. Instead it is the animal owner's character and preferences that must be called to account for a population-wide problem that crosses class structures, cultures, and for those animals who live amongst us, it would seem, species. As a point of reflection on how we conceptualize intersections and interactions between human and companion health and welfare, if news-reporting conveys information that ordinary people apply to themselves and those around them, individualizing culpability for canine obesity may have broader political effects. At a time when public health researchers struggle to raise the public profile of structural influences on weight-related problems in human populations, this evolving "animal story" may reinforce the notion that excess weight in owners, their pet animals, or both, is indicative of a personal failure and low moral worth. In turn, this way of framing suggests that the only solution is to call for greater individual discipline, which, if needed, can be aided by a clinically orientated intervention.

Acknowledgements

We thank Lorraine Toews, Liaison Librarian for the Faculty of Veterinary Medicine at the University of Calgary, for her expertise and assistance in compiling the search materials, and the three anonymous reviewers for their insights and suggestions. Chris Degeling is funded by a University of Calgary Veterinary Medicine Entrance Award. Melanie Rock holds a Population Health Investigator award from Alberta Innovates—Health Solutions, which is funded by the Alberta Heritage Foundation for Medical Research Endowment Fund. She also holds a New Investigator award from the Canadian Institutes of Health Research.

References

Altheide, D. L. 1987. Ethnographic content analysis. *Qualitative Sociology* 10: 65–77.

Barry, C. L., Brescoll, V. L., Brownell, K. D. and Schlesinger, M. 2009. Obesity metaphors: How beliefs about the causes of obesity affect support for public policy. *Milbank Quarterly* 87: 7–47.

Bee, P. 2005. Is your pet as podgy as you? *The Times* (UK). July 1, T2, p. 8.

Blue, G. and Rock, M. 2011. in press. Trans-biopolitics: Complexity in interspecies relations. *Health* DOI: 10.1177/1363459310376299.

Borkan, J. 1999. Immersion/crystallization. In *Doing Qualitative Research*, 179–194. ed. B. Crabtree and W. Miller. London: Sage.

Bourdieu, P. 1995. *Outline of a Theory of Practice.* Cambridge: Cambridge University Press.

Brodie, M., Hamel, E. C., Altman, D. E., Blendon, R. J. and Benson, J. M. 2003. Health news and the American public, 1996–2002. *Journal of Health Politics Policy and Law* 28: 927–950.

Coren, A. 2005. Crunchy snacks to avoid: A practical guide to pet care this festive season. *The Times* (UK), December 14, p. 17.

Covic, T., Roufeil, L. and Dziurawiec, S. 2007. Community beliefs about childhood obesity: Its causes, consequences and potential solutions. *Journal of Public Health* 29: 123–131.

Cutt, H., Giles-Corti, B., Knuiman, M. and Burke, V. 2007. Dog ownership, health and physical activity: A critical review of the literature. *Health and Place* 13: 261–272.

Derbyshire, D. 2008. Barking mad: Owners of obese dogs and fat cats could face jail under controversial new rules. Daily Mail (UK): November 4. <www.dailymail.co.uk> Article ID: 1083010.

Dogs don't need diet pills, need disciplined care. 2007. American News (Aberdeen, SD): January 9. <www.aberdeennews.com> Article ID: 116979C662B80020.

Entman, R. M. 1993. Framing: Toward clarification of a fractured paradigm. *The Journal of Communication* 43: 51–58.

Entman, R. M. and Herbst, S. 2001. Reframing public opinion as we have known It. In *Mediated Politics,* 203–225, ed. L. Bennet and R. Entman. Cambridge: Cambridge University Press.

Evans, W. D., Finkelstein, E. A., Kamerow, D. B. and Renaud, J. M. 2005. Public perceptions of childhood obesity. *American Journal of Preventive Medicine* 28: 26–32.

Fackelmann, K. 2003. It's a dog-eat-too-much world. *USA Today*, October 28, p. 9.

Foresight Report. 2007. *Tackling Obesities: Future Choices–Project Report.* London, UK: Government Office for Science.

Franklin, A. 1999. *Animals and Modern Cultures: A Sociology of Human–Animal Relations in Modernity.* London: Sage.

Franklin, A. and White, R. 2001. Animals and modernity: Changing human–animal relationships, 1949–98. *Journal of Sociology* 37: 219–238.

Gardiner, A. 2009. The animal as surgical patient: A historical perspective in the 20th century. *History and Philosophy of the Life Sciences* 31: 355–376.

Hamilton, A. 2004. Even poor old Fido's fighting the flab. *The Times* (UK). October 18, p. 9.

Harper, J. 2007. Corpulent canines prove bark imitates life. Washington Times, The (DC). January 28. <www.washingtontimes.com> Article ID: 5200701280334370010042.

Hughes, H. M. 1940. *News and the Human Interest Story.* Chicago, IL: The University of Chicago Press.

James, W. P. 2008. The epidemiology of obesity: The size of the problem. *Journal of Internal Medicine* 263: 336–352.

Kersh, R. and Morone, J. A. 2005. Obesity, courts, and the new politics of public health. *Journal of Health Politics Policy and Law* 30: 839–868.

Krippendorff, K. 2004. *Content Analysis: An Introduction to its Methodology.* Thousand Oaks, CA: Sage.

Lallo, M. 2007. Fat? Not me, I'm just big-boned: Now pets are set for a diet pill. The Age (Australia): January 14. <www.theage.com.au> Article ID: 1168105227873.

Lawrence, R. G. 2004. Framing obesity. *The Harvard International Journal of Press/Politics* 9: 56–75.

LeCompte, M. and Schensul, J. 1999. *Analyzing and Interpreting Ethnographic Data.* Walnut Creek, CA: AltaMira Press.

Lund, E. M., Armstrong, P. J., Kirk, C. A. and Klausner, J. S. 2006. Prevalence and risk factors for obesity in adult dogs from private US veterinary practices. *International Journal of Applied Research in Veterinary Medicine* 4: 177–186.

Maziak, W., Ward, K. D. and Stockton, M. B. 2008. Childhood obesity: Are we missing the big picture? *Obesity Reviews* 9: 35–42.

McGreevy, P. D., Thomson, P. C., Pride, C., Fawcett, A., Grassi, T. and Jones, B. 2005. Prevalence of obesity in dogs examined by Australian veterinary practices and the risk factors involved. *Veterinary Record* 156: 695–702.

McLaren, L. 2007. Socioeconomic status and obesity. *Epidemiologic Reviews* 29: 29–48.

Menzer, K. 2007. Key to pet weight gain lies in owners' hands. *The Dallas Morning News:* January 9. <www.dallasnews.com>.

Miller, D. 1998. *A Theory of Shopping.* Ithaca, NY: Cornell University Press.

Morgan, K. 2006. Fat cats & jumbo dogs: Pet obesity rising but stoppable if owners can say no. The Charleston Gazette: September 26. <www.wvgazette.com>.

Moscovici, S. 2000. *Social Representations.* Cambridge, UK: Polity Press.

Mykhalovskiy, E. 2003. Evidence-based medicine: Ambivalent reading and the clinical recontextualization of science. *Health* 7: 331–352.

National Research Council: Committee on Animal Nutrition. 2003. Publication Announcement: New Dietary Guidelines Issued for Cats and Dogs. Office of News and Public Information. National Academy of Sciences <http://www.nationalacademies.org/onpinews/newsitem.aspx?> Record ID = 10668.

Nijland, M. L., Stam, F. and Seidell, J. C. 2010. Overweight in dogs, but not in cats, is related to overweight in their owners. *Public Health Nutrition* 13: 102–106.

Oliver, J. E. and Lee, T. 2005. Public opinion and the politics of obesity in America. *Journal of Health Politics Policy and Law* 30: 923–954.

Our doggies, ourselves. 2006. *St. Louis Post-Dispatch* (MO), February 27, p. D10.

Podberscek, A. L. 1994. Dog on a tightrope: The position of the dog in British society as influenced by press reports on dog attacks (1988 to 1992). *Anthrozoös* 7: 232–241.

Porky pets. 2003. *New York Times.* September 15, p. 18.

Potestio, M., McLaren, L., Robinson Vollman, A. and Doyle-Baker, P. 2008. Childhood obesity: Perceptions held by the public in Calgary, Canada. *Canadian Journal of Public Health* 99: 86–90.

Rail, G., Holmes, D. and Murray, S. 2010. The politics of evidence on "domestic terrorists": Obesity discourses and their effects. *Social Theory & Health* 8: 259–279.

Rohlf, V. I., Toukhsati, S., Coleman, G. J. and Bennett, P. C. 2010. Dog obesity: Can dog caregivers' (owners') feeding and exercise intentions and behaviors be predicted from attitudes? *Journal of Applied Animal Welfare Science* 13: 213–236.

Saguy, A. C. and Almeling, R. 2008. Fat in the fire? Science, the news media, and the "Obesity Epidemic." *Sociological Forum* 23: 53–83.

Sexton, K. 2004. Epidemic of obese pets. *The Sunday Telegraph* (Australia). November 28. p. L34.

Skotnicki, K. 2004. Obesity dogs pets. *Sunday Herald Sun* (Australia): December 5, p. 32.

Smith, D. E. 1999. *Writing the Social: Critique, Theory, and Investigations.* Toronto: University of Toronto Press.

Tester, K. 1991. *Animals and Society: The Humanity of Animal Rights.* London: Routledge.

Trumble, T. 2006. Pets going to the dogs. *Herald Sun* (Australia), June 30, p. 35.

Turner, J. 1980. *Reckoning with the Beast: Animals, Pain, and Humanity in the Victorian Mind.* Baltimore, MD: Johns Hopkins University.

US Department of Health and Human Services. 2001. The Surgeon General's Call to Action to Prevent and Decrease Overweight and Obesity. Rockville, MD: US Department of Health and Human Services: Public Health Service, Office of the Surgeon General.

Viner, R. M., Roche, E., Maguire, S. A. and Nicholls, D. E. 2010. Childhood protection and obesity: Framework for practice. 47341: c3074.

Wang, Z. and Gantz, W. 2007. Health content in local television news. *Health Communication* 21: 213–221.

Washer, P. 2004. Representations of SARS in the British newspapers. *Social Science & Medicine* 59: 2561–2571.

Washer, P. 2006. Representations of mad cow disease. *Social Science & Medicine* 62: 457–466.

Washer, P. and Joffe, H. 2006. The "hospital superbug": Social representations of MRSA. *Social Science & Medicine* 63: 2141–2152.

ANTHROZOÖS VOLUME 25, ISSUE 1 REPRINTS AVAILABLE PHOTOCOPYING © ISAZ 2012
 PP. 49–60 DIRECTLY FROM PERMITTED PRINTED IN THE UK
  THE PUBLISHERS BY LICENSE ONLY

A Survey of Pet- and Non-Pet-Owning Swedish Adolescents: Demographic Differences and Health Issues

Maria Müllersdorf*, Fredrik Granström† and Per Tillgren*‡

*Mälardalen University, School of Health, Care and Social Welfare, Eskilstuna/Västerås, Sweden

†R&D Centre/Centre for Clinical Research, Sörmland County Council, Eskilstuna, Sweden

‡Karolinska Institute, Department of Public Health Sciences, Stockholm, Sweden

Address for correspondence:
Maria Müllersdorf,
Mälardalen University,
School of Health, Care and
Social Welfare,
PO Box 325, SE-631 05
Eskilstuna, Sweden.
E-mail:
maria.mullersdorf@mdh.se

ABSTRACT The aim of this study was to describe the prevalence of pet ownership in adolescents in Sweden and establish whether any gender, age or health-related differences exist between those who own pets and those who do not. In addition, the study aimed to explore the relationships between species of pet, age, gender, and other socio-demographic variables and the perceived importance of pets. Three age groups (13–14 years-old, 15–16 years-old, and 17–18 years-old) of adolescents, resident in a single county in Sweden, were surveyed using the questionnaire "Liv och Hälsa Ung" ("Youth Life and Health"). A total of 8,709 respondents were included in the analysis (pet owners = 5,793; non-pet owners = 2,916). Associations between importance of the pet and demographic variables and general self-rated health were investigated using logistic regression analysis. The prevalence of pet owners in the sample was 65%, and the most common types of pets were, in descending order of popularity, cats, dogs, rodents, fish/reptiles, and horses. Most of the pet owners said their pets were very or quite important to them, for the three age groups (73.1–88.6%). In general, pets were more important for the female respondents. Importance was dependent on type of pet, with male and female dog owners and female horse owners rating their pets as more important than the owners of other species of pet. Respondents who did not own a pet were more physically active than their pet-owning peers. Pet owners with the best self-rated health also attributed the greatest importance to their pet. However, adolescents with pets reported more psychological problems and somatic health aspects than those who did not own pets. This finding calls for further studies to be conducted, with designs allowing causal conclusions to be drawn.

Anthrozoös DOI: 10.2752/175303712X13240472427276

Keywords: adolescents, health, pets, prevalence, Sweden

The prevalence of pets is high in Western society. In Sweden, 12.8% of households have dogs, 16.8% have cats, and 9.5% have other types of pet. Households with children/adolescents have a higher rate of pet ownership than those without children: 19.3% for dogs and 22.5% for cats (Statistics Sweden 2006). A study of adolescents aged 12–17 years in the USA identified that 50% of adolescents were pet owners, and that some socio-demographic characteristics were positively associated with pet ownership, such as race (Caucasian), income (higher), and living circumstance (single-family home). The importance of the pet was rated highest among white adolescents without siblings, families with moderate income or above, and dog or cat owners (Siegel 1995). In America, Australia, and the United Kingdom, dogs are common in families with children (≤ 11 years) and adolescents (12–19 years) (Westgarth et al. 2007). Pet ownership has been found to vary with certain socio-economic conditions, such as the presence of children or adolescents in the household (Westgarth et al. 2007) and immigrant status (Klumpers and Endenburg 2009). However, to our knowledge, no studies have explored the prevalence of pet ownership among adolescents, or their relationship with their pets, in a general European population. Further, previous studies have only considered broad age ranges, for example, 6–19 years (Westgarth et al. 2007) and 12–17 years (Siegel 1995).

Children's relationships with pets as special friends or as important family members, and as sources of emotional support, have been reported (Bryant 1990; Triebenbacher 1998). The relationship between a child and pet can serve as a protective factor for children experiencing inter-parental conflict (Strand 2004), resulting in children in single-parent families bonding more strongly with their dog than do those in two-parent families (Bodsworth and Coleman 2001). It has also been argued that a dog may serve as a substitute companion or even a parental substitute (Archer 1997).

Health has generally improved in the Swedish population since the Second World War (National Swedish Board of Health and Welfare 2009). However, since 1990, young people between 16 and 24 years of age have not shown the same positive development as other age groups, especially with regard to psychological health in women. Self-reported anxiety and worry increased from 8 to 29% among young women and from 2 to 7% among young men between 1988–1989 and 2004–2005. A representative Swedish national study of adolescents aged 11, 13, and 15 years identified that the rate of psychological problems increases with age and is higher among females compared with males (Swedish National Board for Youth Affairs 2007). This pattern is also seen in older (16–24 years) Swedish females (Swedish National Institute of Public Health 2006).

Studies have shown that having contact with a pet has a positive impact on well-being, perception of loneliness (Banks and Banks 2002), depression (Dembicki and Anderson 1996), and general health (Raina et al. 1999), especially for those who form a bond with their pet (Cutt et al. 2007). Most of these studies concern specific groups, such as elderly people or people with disabilities. The benefits of the human–companion animal bond have been reported (Friedmann and Son 2009), but the type of relationship between pet and owner is also important. Studies of compatibility— the match between the pet and the owner—measured on health dimensions, show that a higher degree of compatibility between pet and owner is associated with better-reported psychological health and fewer symptoms of physical ill-health (Budge et al. 1998). The association between the bond between human and pet and its relationship with blood pressure has also been investigated (Baun et al. 1983), with the greater physical effect displayed if there was an established bond. A direct relationship exists between how people perceive animals and their resulting physiological response to them, with a positive perception resulting in greater physiological benefit to the person than to those with a negative perception (Friedmann, Locker and Lockwood 1993).

Studies based on national general populations have confirmed the positive effects of owning a pet. Pet owners visit the doctor less often (Heady and Grabka 2007), but negative health indicators have also been reported, such as increased depressive symptoms among pet owners compared with non-pet owners (Parslow et al. 2005). Both positive and negative aspects of health were found in a recent Swedish study, based on a large regional population in the age range 18 to 84 years (Müllersdorf et al. 2010). Pet owners had better self-reported general health but suffered more from mental health problems than non-pet owners. Other differences between these groups include pet owners being more likely to be female, younger, and living in a home they owned. Pet owners more often performed moderate to vigorous intense exercise (five hours or more/week), whereas non-pet owners more often performed light exercise (less than two hours/week).

In sum, previous studies have demonstrated relationships between pet ownership and physical and mental health and exercise levels in the Western world. However, we have not found comparable studies concerning adolescents. The prevalence and perceived importance of pets among adolescents in a general population in Europe seems also to be unexplored. While age and gender differences between pet owners and non-pet owners have been identified in adults Swedes (Müllersdorf et al. 2010), it is unknown whether these exist in adolescents.

Aims

The aims of this study were to gather data on the prevalence of pet ownership, health-related variables, and the perceived importance of pets among adolescents in Sweden, and determine whether any relationships exist between these variables including socio-demographic aspects.

Methods
Participants and Procedure

Adolescents aged 13–14 years, 15–16 years, and 17–18 years from a central Sweden local-government area were invited to participate in a survey which was conducted in school classrooms in 2008. Questionnaires were returned in sealed envelopes to ensure confidentiality.

All of the schools ($n = 65$) in the county of Södermanland were invited to participate and 62 agreed (the three non-participating schools were small, with fewer than 30 students in each age group). In 2008, the total number of inhabitants in the age range (13–19 years) in the county was 11,073. A total of 10,680 adolescents (aged 13–14 years = 3,353; aged 15–16 years = 3,740; aged 17–18 years = 3,587) were surveyed, resulting in a response rate of 83% ($n = 8,891$; aged 13–14 years = 2,951; aged 15–16 years = 3,142; aged 17–18 years = 2,798).

Questionnaire Design

The questionnaire, "Liv och Hälsa Ung" ("Youth Life and Health"), encompassed items that were grouped into various categories: demographics, health, school, life habits, tobacco and alcohol, violence, road safety, leisure time, and security/participation (in total, 68 items). In addition, items aimed specifically at the age groups 15–16 years and 17–18 years were included in the following areas: guidance centers for young people, drugs, love/sex/coexistence, and criminality (giving an overall total of 96 items). For the current study, the fourteen items chosen for analysis were: demographics (sex [1], housing [3], native country [1]), health (general [1], physical [2] and mental [3]), life habits (pet ownership [1] and importance of the pet [1]), and leisure time (physical activity [1]). The pet-ownership item asked respondents to identify which species they owned and provided the following species options: cat, dog, rabbit, guinea pig/hamster/rat, aquarium fish, reptile, horse, and other.

Data Analysis

The Statistical Package for the Social Sciences (SPSS) 17.0 (Chicago, IL, USA) was used for all analyses. The significance level was set at < 0.05. A total of 8,709 (81.5% of the respondents: 2,900 aged 13–14 years; 3,048 aged 15–16 years, and 2,761 aged 17–18 years) answered the question whether they had a pet or not (5,793 [66.5%] had a pet and 2,916 [33.5%] did not). Differences between male and female students, between those who owned pets and those who did not, and between age groups were explored using chi-square statistics. Logistic regression analysis was performed to calculate the odds ratios (ORs) for rating a pet as very important, based on the question "How important is your pet/pets to you?" with four possible responses: "Very important," "Quite important," "Not very important," and "Not important at all." Models were created to predict the odds of a "Very important" response being given by contrast with any of the other possible responses, based on the following independent variables: type of pet, age group, family situation, and self-rated general health. Separate models were fitted for males and females.

Results

Socio-Demographics

Significantly greater proportions of pet-owning participants were "home owners" and born in Sweden than those who did not own a pet. Significantly more students who lived with both parents were non-pet owners, whereas adolescents with alternating living circumstances (living in turn with one parent for a time, then with the other) were more often pet owners (see Table 1).

Prevalence of Pets

The prevalence of pet owners among the adolescents is displayed in Table 2. Overall, the prevalence of pets was 66.5%, with cats most common (33%, $n = 3,239$), followed by dogs (26.6%, $n = 2,608$). The third most common type of pet was rodents (15.6%, $n = 1,532$), followed by fish/reptiles (10.1%, $n = 990$) and horses (7.5%, $n = 736$). The distribution was consistent across age groups. The prevalence of dogs increased from the 13–16 years age group to the 15–16 years age group and of cats from the 13–14 years age group to the 17–18 years age group. A decrease in the numbers of rodents, fish/reptiles, and horses from the 13–14 years age group to the 17–18 years age group was detected. More than a third of the pet owners (37.7%, $n = 2,181$) had more than one pet—a proportion that was constant across age groups. Generally, prevalence of pet ownership was higher among females. Details of prevalence for each type of pet by each age group and gender are presented in Table 2.

Aspects of Health

Differences between pet owners and non-pet owners were detected concerning aspects of health. A significantly greater proportion of pet owners in all three age groups reported feeling "not good," as well as having stomach ache and feeling depressed, compared with non-pet owners. Pet owners from the 13–14 years age group also experienced headache, difficulties in falling asleep, and feeling stressed more often than non-pet owners of the same ages. Pet

Table 1. Socio-demographic variables of the adolescents by pet ownership and age group.

Item	Response Option	Group[1]	Pet Owner (%)	Non-Pet Owner (%)	χ^2
Sex	Male	1	46.7	60.1	
(n = 8,692)	Female		53.3	39.9	45.55***
	Male	2	46.7	53.4	
	Female		53.3	46.6	11.98**
	Male	3	48.2	57.7	
	Female		51.8	42.3	22.69***
Living in More	Yes	1	28.1	19.2	
Than One Place	No		71.9	80.8	26.60***
(n = 8,657)	Yes	2	29.8	22.2	
	No		70.2	77.8	19.82***
	Yes	3	31.1	20.7	
	No		68.9	79.3	33.94***
Housing	Rented apartment	1	11.9	27.7	
(n = 8,675)	Owned apartment/house		87.0	71.2	
	Other		1.1	1.1	110.42***
	Rented apartment	2	11.3	28.1	
	Owned apartment/house		87.6	71.3	
	Other		1.1	0.6	136.80***
	Rented apartment	3	15.9	29.4	
	Owned apartment/house		83.8	70.2	
	Other		0.2	0.4	70.76***
Lives Together	Both mother and father	1	61.3	68.3	
with	Single parent		6.9	8.8	
(n = 8,642)	One parent and his/her partner		4.6	2.6	
	Alternating living condition[2]		22.8	15.0	
	Other		4.5	5.2	33.93***
	Both mother and father	2	57.8	63.0	
	Single parent		8.7	12.2	
	One parent and his/her partner		6.7	5.5	
	Alternating living condition		22.2	16.0	
	Other		4.6	3.3	28.19***
	Both mother and father	3	53.5	63.4	
	Single parent		10.9	12.4	
	One parent and his/her partner		6.9	4.4	
	Alternating living condition		18.1	13.1	
	Other		10.7	6.7	39.02***
Native Country	Swedish	1	93.5	71.1	
(n = 8,527)	European		1.5	5.8	
	Non-European		3.1	21.2	302.84***
	Swedish	2	94.4	75.9	
	European		1.4	5.1	
	Non-European		1.7	15.8	269.79***
	Swedish	3	94.2	76.5	
	European		1.4	4.9	
	Non-European		1.8	16.1	234.70***

[1]Group 1 = aged 13–14 years; Group 2 = aged 15–16 years; Group 3 = aged 17–18 years.

[2]Living in turn with one parent for a time, then with the other.

**p < 0.01, ***p < 0.001.

Table 2. Prevalence of pets, and species of, by age group and gender of owner.

	Group 1 (n = 2,900)[1]				Group 2 (n = 3,048)				Group 3 (n = 2,761)			
	Male	Female	Total[2]	%	Male	Female	Total[2]	%	Male	Female	Total[2]	%
Pet Owners	916	1,046	1,972	68.0	953	1,087	2,043	67.0	857	920	1,778	64.4
Cats	509	542	1,058	30.7	522	590	1,114	33.2	498	568	1,067	37.5
Dogs	392	427	824	24.1	438	522	961	28.6	422	401	823	28.9
Rodents	227	366	600	17.5	169	296	466	13.9	123	196	319	11.2
Fish/Reptiles	169	214	387	11.3	145	198	345	10.3	107	151	258	9.1
Horses	85	164	251	7.3	81	181	263	7.8	59	163	222	7.8
Other Pets	197	118	315	9.2	103	119	222	6.6	74	86	160	5.6
Total No. Pets	1,579	1,831	3,435		1,452	1,906	3,358		1,283	1,565	2,848	
Mean No. Pets	1.72	1.75	1.74		1.52	1.75	1.64		1.49	1.70	1.60	

[1]Group 1 = aged 13–14 years; Group 2 = aged 15–16 years; Group 3 = aged 17–18 years.

[2]A small number of respondents where gender was not specified are included. Thus, the number of males and females does not always exactly sum to the totals.

Table 3. Perception of health and level of physical activity of the adolescents by age group and pet ownership.

Item	Response Option	Group[1]	Pet Owner (%)	Non-Pet Owner (%)	χ^2
How do	Very good	1	48.5	58.2	
you feel?	Good		37.0	32.0	
	Not good		14.5	9.8	26.50***
	Very good	2	37.0	42.3	
	Good		43.3	42.6	
	Not good		19.8	15.0	13.43**
	Very good	3	29.5	38.5	
	Good		52.1	49.2	
	Not good		18.4	12.2	31.27***
How often do	Never or seldom	1	38.4	45.5	
you have a	Once a month		32.7	31.3	
headache?	Once a week/more often		28.8	23.2	15.19**
	Never or seldom	2	31.8	33.3	
	Once a month		32.6	35.0	
	Once a week/more often		35.6	31.7	4.58
	Never or seldom	3	34.2	37.2	
	Once a month		30.2	32.6	
	Once a week/more often		35.6	30.2	7.99*
How often do	Never or seldom	1	51.9	57.9	
you have a	Once a month		32.2	29.2	
stomach ache?	Once a week/more often		15.9	12.9	9.56**
	Never or seldom	2	45.7	49.1	
	Once a month		32.1	33.4	
	Once a week/more often		22.2	17.5	8.89*
	Never or seldom	3	47.8	55.6	
	Once a month		29.9	29.7	
	Once a week/more often		22.2	14.7	25.36***
How often do you	Never or seldom	1	45.1	51.9	
have difficulties	Once a month		24.7	23.8	
in falling asleep?	Once a week/more often		30.2	24.3	14.04**
	Never or seldom	2	39.8	40.3	
	Once a month		21.2	22.9	
	Once a week/ more often		39.1	36.7	1.97
	Never or seldom	3	37.3	37.3	
	Once a month		23.6	24.5	
	Once a week/more often		39.2	38.2	0.41

[1]Group 1 = aged 13–14 years; Group 2 = aged 15–16 years; Group 3 = aged 17–18 years.

*$p < 0.05$, **$p < 0.01$, ***$p < 0.001$.

Table 4. Importance of pets and species of pet by age group and gender of owner.

		Male Owners n (%)			Female Owners n (%)		
Group[1]		Not Important	Quite Important	Very Important	Not Important	Quite Important	Very Important
1	Pet owners	122 (13.5)	266 (29.5)	513 (56.9)	76 (7.3)	201 (19.4)	759 (73.3)
	Cats	47 (9.4)	150 (29.9)	305 (60.8)	27 (5.0)	90 (16.8)	420 (70.4)
	Dogs	20 (5.2)	93 (24.3)	270 (70.5)	10 (2.4)	51 (12.0)	364 (85.6)
	Rodents	34 (15.2)	74 (33.0)	116 (51.8)	14 (3.9)	71 (19.7)	276 (76.5)
	Fish/reptiles	41 (24.7)	46 (27.7)	79 (47.6)	34 (16.2)	41 (19.5)	135 (64.3)
	Horses	10 (11.9)	29 (34.5)	45 (53.6)	4 (2.5)	19 (11.7)	140 (85.9)
2	Pet owners	228 (24.1)	312 (33.0)	406 (42.9)	119 (11.0)	220 (20.3)	743 (68.7)
	Cats	99 (19.1)	190 (36.7)	229 (44.2)	35 (5.9)	109 (18.5)	445 (75.6)
	Dogs	64 (14.7)	139 (32.0)	231 (53.2)	33 (6.4)	90 (17.4)	395 (76.3)
	Rodents	64 (37.9)	50 (29.6)	55 (32.5)	39 (13.3)	83 (28.3)	171 (58.4)
	Fish/reptiles	52 (36.1)	39 (27.1)	53 (36.8)	40 (20.3)	40 (20.3)	117 (59.4)
	Horses	23 (28.8)	23 (28.8)	34 (42.5)	8 (4.4)	19 (10.5)	154 (85.1)
3	Pet owners	223 (26.1)	311 (36.4)	320 (37.5)	104 (11.4)	185 (20.2)	625 (68.4)
	Cats	113 (22.7)	199 (40.0)	185 (37.2)	39 (6.9)	109 (19.3)	417 (73.8)
	Dogs	64 (15.3)	147 (35.1)	208 (49.6)	18 (4.5)	75 (18.7)	308 (76.8)
	Rodents	50 (41.0)	37 (30.3)	35 (28.7)	28 (14.4)	37 (19.1)	129 (66.5)
	Fish/reptiles	46 (43.4)	32 (30.2)	28 (26.4)	33 (21.9)	23 (15.2)	95 (62.9)
	Horses	20 (33.9)	21(35.6)	18 (30.5)	3 (1.9)	21 (13.0)	138 (85.2)

[1]Group 1 = aged 13–14 years; Group 2 = aged 15–16 years; Group 3 = aged 17–18 years.

owners from the 13–14 years and 17–18 years age groups reported being physically active fewer times per week than non-pet owners.

Importance of the Pet

Adolescents regarded their pets generally as either very or quite important; however, importance ratings for most pets decreased with age. The highest importance ratings were recorded in the 13–14 years age group (males = 86.5%; females = 92.7%), lower levels in the 15–16 years age group (males = 75.9%; females = 89.0%), and the lowest levels were recorded in the 17–18 years age group (males = 73.9%; females = 88.6%). Female students who owned horses mostly rated these animals as being important to them, with rates of 95.6–98.2%, irrespective of age group, higher than adolescents with other types of pets (Table 4).

Using a multivariate logistic regression analysis to determine the Odds Ratios (OR), we found that dog owners perceived their pets as very important more often than cat owners. Adolescents who owned rodents or fish/reptiles were less likely than cat owners to rate their pet as very important. There was a strong gender difference apparent in horse owners, with male horse owners relatively unlikely (OR = 0.69), to rate their pet as very important compared with female horse owners (OR = 2.53). Interestingly, this value was greater than the OR obtained for dog owners (males OR = 2.42; females OR = 2.02).

It is apparent from Table 5 that older participants rated pets as significantly less important than younger ones. This effect was less pronounced among females, particularly amongst

Table 5. Multivariate logistic regression predicting pet owners' probability of rating their pet as very important to them ($n = 5,668$).

Predictor	Male Owners			Female Owners		
	OR	SE	β	OR	SE	β
Species of Pet						
Cats	1.00	(ref)	–	1.00	(ref)	–
Dogs	2.42	0.88	0.08***	2.02	0.70	0.09***
Rodents	0.75	–0.28	0.11**	0.81	–0.21	0.09*
Fish/reptiles	0.67	–0.40	0.12**	0.61	–0.49	0.10***
Horses	0.69	–0.38	0.15*	2.53	0.93	0.14***
Groups						
13–14 years old	1.00	(ref)	–	1.00	(ref)	–
15–16 years old	0.52	–0.66	0.10***	0.74	–0.30	0.10**
17–18 years old	0.40	–0.92	0.10***	0.72	–0.33	0.11**
Household Composition						
Both mother and father	1.00	(ref)	–	1.00	(ref)	–
Single parent	0.95	–0.06	0.15	1.06	0.06	0.15
One parent and his/her partner	0.93	–0.08	0.17	0.96	–0.04	0.18
Alternating living condition[1]	1.05	0.05	0.10	0.72	–0.34	0.10**
Other	1.03	0.03	0.19	0.98	–0.02	0.17
How Do You Feel?						
Good	1.00	(ref)	–	1.00	(ref)	–
Very good	1.24	0.22	0.09*	1.35	0.30	0.10**
Not good	1.01	0.01	0.11	0.90	–0.11	0.10

[1]Living in turn with one parent for a time, then with the other.

$*p < 0.05$, $**p < 0.01$, $***p < 0.001$.

older, female horse owners. There was little relationship between the perceived importance of a pet and household composition. The only significant OR in relation to the reference group—those living with both mother and father—was found for females living alternately with separated parents (OR = 0.72, $p = 0.001$), where pets were less likely to be rated as very important. The probability of rating the pet as very important was higher among males (OR = 1.24, $p = 0.01$) and females (OR = 1.35, $p = 0.003$) with very good self-rated health.

Discussion

The aims of this study were to gather data on the prevalence of pet ownership, health-related variables, and the perceived importance of pets among adolescents in Sweden, and determine whether any relationships exist between these variables.

Two-thirds of adolescents in this study owned a pet, with the prevalence decreasing with age. Swedish national figures for households with children/adolescents (aged 0–18 years) identify that 19.3% have dogs and 22.5% cats (Statistics Sweden 2006), which is lower than that found in this study (dogs 26.6%; cats 33.0%). However, our sample included adolescents aged 13–18 years, and is therefore not fully comparable with the national data. Also, a higher prevalence of pets is found in counties situated outside metropolitan areas in Sweden (Statistics

Sweden 2006), which was the case for our sample. Nevertheless, this study confirms previous results from other countries that pets are common in families with children/adolescents (West-garth et al. 2007). Similar to findings from the Netherlands (Klumpers and Endenburg 2009), pet owners tended to be native-born (Swedes in this case), with immigrants owning fewer pets. Cats were the most common type of pet, followed by dogs and rodents, which is in line with the reported prevalence of pets in Sweden in 2006 (Swedish Kennel Club 2007).

Adolescents generally rated the importance of their pets highly, with the importance of the pet decreasing with age. Females consistently rated their pets as more important than males of the same age, except when dogs were the pets owned. This agrees with previous reports of species differences in how people rate various species of pet (Siegel 1995). However, we did not find any connection between importance of the pet and not living with both mother and father. In this study, the adolescents with pets more often lived under what we have called alternating circumstances compared with those without pets, verifying Siegels' 1995 study. Interestingly, female adolescents living under alternating circumstances were the ones who least often stated that their pet was very important to them.

More negative health signs were reported by pet owners compared with non-pet owners, as was the case in a recent study of Swedish adults (Müllersdorf et al. 2010). Both studies found that pet owners reported more psychological problems than non-pet owners. Among adolescents in Sweden, psychosomatic health complaints increased between 1988 and 2005 (Hagquist 2009), but there are no explanations for why adolescents with pets might report more psychological problems than their peers without pets. Maybe, people with psychologi-cal problems, irrespective of age, tend to get a pet in the hope of reducing loneliness and/or obtaining social support in the form of a loving but non-demanding companion. The associ-ation between pet ownership and reports of psychological problems is likely to be complex, and interpretations should therefore be made with caution. However, by contrast with pet-owning adults, the proportion with good self-rated general health was lower among pet-owning adolescents compared with adolescents without pets (Müllersdorf et al. 2010). This supports the finding that 16–24-year-olds do not show the same positive health trends as other Swedes, particularly regarding psychological health (National Swedish Board of Health and Welfare 2009).

Interestingly, and partly in contradiction to the overall negative health picture for adolescents with pets in this study, pet owners with the best self-rated health were the ones attaching the greatest importance to their pet. It is not possible to draw any causal conclusions on the basis of this study, but a productive area for future research might be to investigate whether the strength of feeling adolescents have for their pets promotes better health.

The results showed that young people with pets in the 13–14 years and 17–18 years age groups were less physically active than those who did not own a pet. This is in contrast to find-ings for Swedish adults with pets, who are more physically active in their daily life (Müllersdorf et al 2010). Possibly, adults with pets have formed patterns of physical activity that includes the pet, whereas adolescents are developing towards a lifestyle as grown-ups that may or may not include a pet. This difference concerning physical activity between adults and adolescents with pets is another area for further research.

The ability to generalize from this study is limited due to respondents being recruited from a single county in Sweden. However, the large and comprehensive sample and high response rate should provide representative data for that region. A questionnaire always has limitations, including how truthfully respondents reply to the items. This was mitigated, to some extent, by allowing students to respond anonymously. The study's limitations lie mainly in its retrospective design and the limited number of items concerning pet ownership and its related importance. Since just a single item was used to measure the importance of a pet, there is a risk of mono-method bias (Cook and Campbell 1979). In this case, the survey was being used for multiple purposes, and the researchers were only allowed to include two additional questions regarding pets (one concerning prevalence, the other importance). Future similar studies should utilize a pet attachment scale.

In conclusion, adolescents who owned pets reported greater negative personal health than those without pets, a finding that calls for further studies, ones with designs allowing causal conclusions to be drawn.

Acknowledgements

The study was financially supported by Mälardalen University and Sörmland County Council.

References

Archer, J. 1997. Why do people love their pets? *Evolution and Human Behavior* 18: 237–259.

Banks, M. R. and Banks, W. A. 2002. The effects of animal-assisted therapy on loneliness in an elderly population in long-term care facilities. *Journal of Gerontology: Medical Sciences* 57: 428–432.

Baun M. M., Bergstrom, N., Langston, N. F. and Thoma, L. 1983. Physiological effects of human/companion animal bonding. *Nursing Research* 33: 126–129.

Bodsworth, W. and Coleman, G. J. 2001. Child–companion animal attachment bonds in single and two-parent families. *Anthrozoös* 14: 216–223.

Bryant, B. K. 1990. The richness of the child–pet relationship: A consideration of both benefits and costs of pets to children. *Anthrozoös* 3: 253–261.

Budge, R. C., Spicer, J., Jones, B. and St. George, R. 1998. Health correlates of compatibility and attachment in human–companion animal relationships. *Society & Animals* 6: 219–234.

Cook, T. D. and Campbell, D. T. 1979. *Quasi-Experimentation: Design & Analysis Issues for Field Settings.* Boston, MA: Houghton Mifflin.

Cutt, H., Giles-Corti, B., Knuiman, M. and Burke, V. 2007. Dog ownership, health and physical activity: A critical review of the literature. *Health & Place* 13: 261–272.

Dembicki, D. and Anderson, K. 1996. Pet ownership may be a factor in improved health of the elderly. *Journal of Nutrition for the Elderly* 15: 15–31.

Friedmann, E., Locker B. Z. and Lockwood, R. 1993. Perception of animals and cardiovascular responses during verbalization with an animal present. *Anthrozoös* 6: 115–134.

Friedmann, E. and Son, H. 2009. The human–companion animal bond: How humans benefit. *Veterinary Clinics of North America* 39: 293–326.

Hagquist, C. 2009. Psychosomatic health problems among adolescents in Sweden—are the time trends gender related? *European Journal of Public Health* 19: 331–336.

Heady, B. and Grabka, M. M. 2007. Pets and human health in Germany and Australia: *National longitudinal results. Social Indicators Research* 80: 207–311.

Klumpers, M. and Endenburg, N. 2009. Pets, veterinarians, and multicultural society. *Tijdschrift voor Diergeneeskunde* 134: 54–61.

Müllersdorf, M., Granström, F., Sahlqvist, L. and Tillgren, P. 2010. Aspects of health, physical/leisure activities, work and socio-demographics associated with pet ownership in Sweden. *Scandinavian Journal of Public Health* 38: 53–63.

National Swedish Board of Health and Welfare. 2009. *Folkhälsorapport* 2009. (Public Health Report 2009). Stockholm: Socialstyrelsen. (in Swedish)

Parslow, R. A., Jorm, A. F., Christensen, H. and Rodgers, B. 2005. Pet ownership and health in older adults: Findings from a survey of 2,551 community-based Australians aged 60–64. *Gerontology* 51: 40–47.

Raina, P., Waltner-Toews, D., Bonnet, B., Woodward, C. and Abernathy, T. 1999. Influence of companion animals on the physical and psychological health of older people: An analysis of a one-year longitudinal study. *Journal of the American Geriatrics Society* 47: 323–329.

Siegel, J. M. 1995. Pet ownership and the importance of pets among adolescents. *Anthrozoös* 7: 217–223.

Statistics Sweden. 2006. Förekomst av sällskapsdjur—främst hund och katt—i svenska hushåll. (Prevalence of pets—mainly dog and cat—in Swedish households). <http://www.manimalis.se/uploads/hela-studieresultatet-sallskapsdjur-i-sverige.pdf> Accessed on January 4, 2010.

Strand, E. B. 2004. Interparental conflict and youth maladjustment: The buffering effects of pets. *Stress, Trauma, and Crisis* 7: 151–168.

Swedish National Board for Youth Affairs. 2007. *Fokus 07. En analys om ungas hälsa och utsatthet*. (Focus 07. An analysis of adolescents' health and exposure). Stockholm: Alfa Print AB. (in Swedish)

Swedish National Institute for Public Health. 2006. *Svenska skolbarns hälsovanor 2005/2006*. (Swedish school children's habits of health 2005/2006). (in Swedish)

The Swedish Kennel Club. 2007. 728,972. *Tidningen Hundsport* 9: 3–17. (in Swedish)

Triebenbacher, S. L. 1998. Pets as transitional objects: Their role in children's emotional development. *Psychological Reports* 82: 191–200.

Westgarth, C., Pinchbeck, G., Bradshaw, J., Dawson, S., Gaskell, R. and Christley, R. 2007. Factors associated with dog ownership and contact with dogs in a UK community. *BMC Veterinary Research* 3: 5. <http://www.ncbi.nlm.nih.gov/pmc/articles/PMC1852100/pdf/1746-6148-3-5.pdf> Accessed on July 24, 2009.

ANTHROZOÖS   VOLUME 25, ISSUE 1   REPRINTS AVAILABLE   PHOTOCOPYING   © ISAZ 2012
PP. 61–74   DIRECTLY FROM   PERMITTED   PRINTED IN THE UK
THE PUBLISHERS   BY LICENSE ONLY

Wandering Cats: Attitudes and Behaviors towards Cat Containment in Australia

Samia R. Toukhsati[*], Emily Young[†], Pauleen C. Bennett[‡] and Grahame J. Coleman[*]

[*]School of Psychology & Psychiatry, Animal Welfare Science Centre, Monash University, Australia

[†]School of Behavioural & Social Science & Humanities, Ballarat University, Australia

[‡]School of Psychological Science, LaTrobe University, Australia

Address for correspondence:
Dr Samia Toukhsati,
School of Psychology &
Psychiatry,
Monash University,
Victoria 3800, Australia.
E-mail:
samia.toukhsati@monash.edu

ABSTRACT Cat containment is a prominent cat management issue in Australia that provokes strong, and sometimes opposing, points of view. The aim of this study was to explore beliefs and attitudes towards containment in cat owner and non-owner groups, and to examine cat containment practices in owners. A random sample of 424 Victorian residents was recruited to complete the Community Attitudes towards Companion Animals Survey by telephone interview. The results showed that, of 142 cat owners, 80% contained their cat to a property at night but only 41.2% contained their cat to a property during the day. For cat owners, beliefs about the importance of cat containment were related to concerns regarding the protection of cats from injury and the protection of native wildlife. Beliefs relating to the importance of cat containment most strongly predicted containment practices. Conversely, findings from non-owners revealed that support for containment was generally linked to concerns regarding protection for wildlife and protection of community members from harm or nuisance behaviors. These findings indicate broad support for cat containment and suggest that education relating to the advantages of suitably enriched containment to protect cats from injury would be worthwhile in regions with cat curfews in place.

Keywords: cat, containment, enrichment, nuisance, wildlife

 While cats remain one of the most popular pets in Australia, there has been an annual decline in the number of household cats of more than 1.5% (Baldock 1999) and a prediction that this trend will continue (Baldock, Alexander and More 2003). This has been attributed to high de-sexing (neutering) rates of domestic cats (around 90%) and an increasingly negative attitude towards cats due to their perceived threat to native wildlife through predation (Chaseling

Anthrozoös   DOI: 10.2752/175303712X13240472427195

2001). For example, Perry's (1999) study of attitudes towards cats in Mount Isa and Brisbane revealed that 67% of the sample reported problems with cats, such as damage to gardens, wildlife predation, noise of fighting cats, and urine spraying. The Department of Sustainability and Environment (DSE) (1999) identified cats as a major threat to native fauna and stated that over 200 million wild animals were killed by domestic, stray, and feral cats (category membership is determined by the extent of reliance of cats on humans; see Jarman and van der Lee 1993) in Victoria each year. The DSE did not, however, distinguish between non-native and native fauna in these statistics. Moreover, despite public opinion, there is scientific uncertainty regarding the extent to which cats threaten native wildlife populations (Lilith et al. 2006). The predation impact of cats on native wildlife appears to be strongly moderated by the environment in which the cat lives and subject to the availability of various species.

Cat containment can reduce the impact of owned cats on native wildlife populations (Calver et al. 2007; Glen and Dickman 2008), minimize fecal pollution of waterways (Dabritz et al. 2006), and reduce the risk of *Toxoplasma gondii* transmission to humans (Dabritz and Conrad 2010). In addition, containment can reduce the likelihood of unwanted feline pregnancies (DSE 1999; Nutter, Levine and Stoskopf 2004), disease contraction such as Feline Immune Deficiency Syndrome (Bernstein 2007), the risk of injury and death from traffic, fighting and dog attacks (Rochlitz 2004), and from acts of cruelty by humans (Munro and Thrusfield 2001).

Nonetheless, management strategies that constrain the natural behaviors of cats, for example, containment, which limits roaming, remain controversial. Little research has been undertaken on the roaming needs of neutered domestic cats; research that examines the extent to which contained environments are suitably enriched to reduce the likelihood of boredom, stress (Rochlitz 2005) and inactivity and/or allow for the expression of natural behaviors (Jones and McGreevy 2007) is needed. Although domestic cats will range over half a hectare if given the opportunity, it is suspected that they are highly flexible in this respect (Bradshaw 1992) and will be content living a confined life as long as other needs, such as opportunities to play, climb, and rest undisturbed, are catered for (DSE 1999; Jongman 2007) and provided they are accustomed to such an environment from an early age (Rochlitz 2005). As such, although the opportunity to engage in natural behaviors is substantially reduced, suitable containment on the part of cat owners, in addition to de-sexing and the provision of an adequate containment environment for domestic cats, may provide a sound welfare outcome.

The DSE (2003) includes containment as a central component of responsible cat ownership; their definition of which emphasizes the protection of native wildlife. Correspondingly, a large proportion of a sample of cat owners and non-owners in Perth were found to agree with the statement that "domestic cats killing wildlife in the suburbs was a problem" and were generally in favor of government cat control legislation (Grayson, Calver and Styles 2002, p. 537). However, the cat owners and non-owners differed in attitudes towards cat control and wildlife. Eighty-seven percent of non-owners were in support of cat containment to protect wildlife, compared with only 48% of owners. Although non-owners (93%) were more in favor of cat legislation than were owners (76%), support from owners was still high. There was only weak support among both owners and non-owners (less than 50% of the sample) for the council having power to introduce cat-free zones. The authors concluded that there was generally strong support in the community for cat control legislation, a conclusion supported by other studies on community attitudes towards cats in Mount Isa and Brisbane (Perry 1999), Magnetic Island (Scriggins and Murray 1997), and Armadale (Lilith et al. 2006).

In Victoria, van de Kuyt (2004) found there was strong support (85%) for cat confinement at night: largely to prevent wildlife predation, to prevent nuisance behavior, and to protect the cat from injury. In relation to the proposal that cats be confined at all times (24-hour confinement) to the property, there was considerably less support (35% of respondents). In general, respondents believed it to be cruel and unnatural to confine a cat for 24 hours to a property, were concerned about the welfare and happiness of cats during confinement, and showed limited understanding of the legal issues relating to confinement. Notably, however, the more respondents reported having been inconvenienced by dogs and/or cats wandering "at large," the more likely they were to support confinement and micro-chipping.

Attitudes and Behavior

Fishbein and Ajzen (1975, p. 6) defined attitudes as "a learned predisposition to respond to an object in a consistently favorable or unfavorable way." The Theory of Planned Behavior proposes that people's behaviors are affected by how they, and their perception of how others, feel about the object concerned. Consequently, attitudes and social norms predict action (Ajzen and Fishbein 1980). Evidence for this theory in the context of human–animal interactions has been presented by Coleman et al. (2003), who found that positive attitudes were associated with more humane handling of pigs and vice versa. Jackson (1996) claimed that irresponsible cat ownership was due to a number of factors, ranging from ignorance of the law to moral protest against legislation, and that changing attitudes was recommended due to the lasting nature of voluntary change. Behavior-change techniques, using incentives and punishments, should be applied in conjunction with attempts to change attitudes.

The aim of this study was to replicate and extend the findings of van de Kuyt (2004) by examining the attitudes and behaviors of Victorian residents towards cat containment. In this context, it was of primary interest to explore whether differences between non-owners (i.e., respondents who did not own cats but may own other pets) and cat owners would emerge. On the basis of past research, the following exploratory hypotheses were developed:

1) That non-owners will report having been disturbed more frequently by wandering cats than cat owners.

2) That non-owners will show a greater preference for 24-hr cat containment and will consider it more important compared with cat owners. In contrast, owners will indicate a preference for night containment.

3) That support for cat containment will primarily relate to concern about wildlife predation in non-owners and possible injury to cats in owners.

4) That beliefs about, and attitudes towards, cats will be related to the importance placed on containment and support for 24-hr containment.

5) That the majority of owners will not provide opportunities for enrichment for their contained cats.

6) That beliefs relating to the importance of cat containment will be related to containment practices.

Methods

Participants and Procedure

Following approval to conduct the research by the Monash University Human Research Ethics Committee, participants were recruited via randomly selected telephone numbers drawn from the Australian White Pages (Market Pro Database). A maximum of three attempts to contact 4,020 potential participants was made. No contact was able to be made with 2,606 individuals and their recruitment was discontinued when the sample quota was achieved. Of the 1414 potential participants contacted by researchers, 30% agreed to participate. The final sample comprised 424 adults (300 female and 124 male) over the age of 18 years residing in rural and non-rural locations in Victoria, Australia. The higher ratio of females to males is not unusual in attitudinal research that examines animal welfare issues (e.g., Verbeke 2002; Verbeke and Vackier 2004).

When a potential participant answered the phone, interviewers introduced themselves and briefly explained the nature of the research and how the data might be used. Interviewers inquired as to whether the potential participant was over the age of 18 years and permanently residing at the address. Having established this, interviewers asked if respondents, or someone else in their household fitting these criteria, would be prepared to participate in the telephone survey, which would take approximately 20 min to complete at a time of their convenience. Experienced telephone interviewers were sourced from *I-View* (Australian Data Collection and Data Management Company) and Monash University. Interviews were conducted during business hours and in the early evening from January to April in 2005.

Materials

The Community Attitudes Towards Companion Animals Survey (CATCAS) (Toukhsati, Bennett and Coleman 2007) was used to canvass the behaviors, beliefs, attitudes, and knowledge relating to issues about cats (such as registration, de-sexing, feeding of semi-owned cats, breeding, containment, wildlife predation, financial investment, and personal responsibility) in cat owners, dog owners, and cat semi-owners.

The CATCAS comprises five sections:

> Section A: 23 forced-choice questions relating to demographic characteristics, such as age, education, employment, residential location, and others.

> Section B: 96 forced-choice questions about beliefs and practices relating to dog ownership, cat ownership, and cat semi-ownership.

> Section C: 11 forced-choice questions about beliefs and practices in relation to companion animal containment.

> Section D: 9 forced-choice questions relating to the prevalence and behaviors of wandering (uncontained) cats in the neighborhood.

> Section E: a series of forced choice and open-ended questions relating to participants' beliefs and attitudes towards companion animals, namely cats and dogs.

Statistical Analyses

Demographic, ownership characteristics, attitudinal, and behavioral data were explored by way of descriptive statistics. Where interval data violated the assumption of normality, comparisons between groups were explored using Mann-Whitney *U* Tests. Comparisons between groups using nominal data were explored using chi-square analyses. Relationships between attitudinal data were explored using Pearson's correlation coefficients. Factors predicting containment behaviors were explored using Forward Binomial Stepwise Logistic Regression. In relation to assumption testing, Tolerance Values were moderate to high and Variance Inflation Factor scores did not exceed 2.5, thereby indicating an absence of multicollinearity. Scatterplots of the independent variables and the logit of the dependent variable revealed a linear relationship. Moreover, the use of reclassified continuous to categorical independent variables in the logistic regression equation revealed a change in the Odds Ratio. Taken together, these visual and statistical analyses indicate that the assumption of linearity was met. No significant interactions emerged in the Models.

Statistical analyses were conducted using the Statistical Package for the Social Sciences (SPSS) 18 (Chicago, IL, USA) and alpha was set at 0.05.

Results
Demographics
All age categories were reasonably well represented, with somewhat higher representation by middle-aged respondents and somewhat lower representation by young adult respondents. Most of the sample was well educated, with over half having completed secondary level education and over a quarter having attained tertiary qualifications. Over 50% of the sample was engaged in full time, part time, or casual employment and most earned up to $50,000 per annum. Frequency data revealed that approximately half of the participants resided in rural locations and the remainder in non-rural locations (see Table 1). Taken together, these demographic data indicate that this sample was characteristic of Australians residing in Victoria in general (Australian Bureau of Statistics 2005a; 2005b).

Companion Animal Ownership
Descriptive statistics revealed that 70% of respondents owned companion animals. Of the entire sample, 33% owned cats, 51% owned dogs 13% owned birds, 4% owned horses, and 10% owned fish.

Cat Ownership
As can be seen in Table 1, with the exception of those residing in rural settings, the proportion of cat owners was similar across each of the residential locations, with approximately 30% of residents from each category indicating that they owned a cat/s. In contrast, over 70% of participants residing in rural locations (+20 acres) indicated ownership of a cat. It can be speculated that these participants engage their cats in rodent control and other related activities associated with rural environments.

In relation to cat acquisition, most were received as a gift (18.3%) or adopted from a friend or family member (16.9%). Many cats were also purchased from an animal rescue center (13.4%), pet shop (9.2%), licensed breeder (7%), or via newspaper advertising (6.3%). Finally, a reasonable proportion of cats were acquired unintentionally (9.2%), "adopted" the owner (9.2%), were found (6.3%), or by "other" means (4.2%).

Prevalence and Attitudes towards Wandering Cats
Sixty-eight percent of respondents indicated that they had "wandering" cats in their neighborhood. Relative to cat owners, a significantly higher proportion of non-owners indicated having seen wandering cats on more occasions ($\chi^2_{(3)} = 16.05$, $n = 262$, $p < 0.001$) and believed

Table 1. Background variables of the participants by cat ownership status.

	Non-Owner		Cat Owner		Total	
	n	%	*n*	%	*n*	%
Age						
18–25 years	23	82.1	5	17.9	28	6.6
26–35 years	31	56.4	24	43.6	55	13.0
36–45 years	48	57.1	36	42.9	84	19.8
46–55 years	69	70.4	29	29.6	98	23.1
56–65 years	48	61.5	30	38.5	78	18.4
66+ years	63	77.8	18	22.2	81	19.1
Education						
No formal schooling	1	0.4	1	0.7	2	0.5
Primary	15	71.4	6	28.6	21	5.0
Secondary	146	62.7	87	37.3	233	55.0
Technical/tertiary	120	71.4	48	28.6	168	39.6
Employment						
Full time	69	63.3	40	36.7	109	25.8
Part time/casual	69	62.7	41	28.9	110	26.0
Unemployed	143	70.1	61	29.9	204	48.2
Salary						
Less than $50K	143	70.4	60	29.6	203	82.2
Less than $90K	21	63.6	12	36.4	33	13.4
$90K +	9	81.8	2	18.2	11	4.5
Residential Location						
Urban (inner city)	16	69.6	7	30.4	23	5.4
Suburban	130	71.4	52	28.6	182	42.9
Regional city	42	71.2	17	28.8	59	13.9
Country town	69	65.1	37	34.9	106	25.0
Semi-rural	17	68.0	8	32.0	25	5.9
Rural	8	27.6	21	72.4	29	6.8
Total	282	66.5	142	33.5	424	100.0

that the cat population was increasing ($\chi^2_{(2)} = 9.42$, $n = 265$, $p < 0.01$). Moreover, significantly fewer cat owners (53.5%), relative to non-owners (66.8%), thought wandering behavior was a nuisance ($\chi^2_{(2)} = 9.90$, $n = 289$, $p < 0.01$). The data showed that a significantly higher proportion of non-owners (62.9%), relative to cat owners (45.8%), supported the humane trapping of wandering cats ($\chi^2_{(2)} = 11.23$, $n = 422$, $p < 0.01$).

Containment

Respondents ($n = 421$) were asked to select from four options as to when they thought cats should be contained to a property: during the day; during the night; 24-hr containment; or not at all. Most non-owners (61.5%) indicated support for 24-hr containment or containment during the night (28.5%). A reverse pattern of results was evident in cat owners, such that most (60%) indicated that cats should be contained during the night and a smaller proportion were

Table 2. Means and standard deviations (*SD*) for beliefs and attitudes towards cats as a function of cat ownership status.

Beliefs and Attitudes		Cat Owner (*n* = 139–142)				Non-Owner (*n* = 279–280)				
		Min	Max	Mean	SD	Min	Max	Mean	SD	p
Importance of Containment	Day	1	5	3.18	1.20	1	5	4.05	1.16	0.001
	Night	1	5	4.54	0.93	1	5	4.75	0.71	0.001
	24 hr	1	5	3.73	1.03	1	5	4.40	0.91	0.001
Attitude towards Cats	General feelings	1	7	6.06	1.38	1	7	4.34	1.83	0.001
Beliefs Relating to Cats	Cats pose a serious threat to native wildlife	1	7	5.69	1.68	1	7	6.12	1.31	0.01
	Cats do not need to roam	1	7	4.30	2.27	1	7	4.51	2.23	>0.05
	Many people own too many cats	1	7	4.03	2.08	1	7	4.81	1.76	0.001
	In general, cats are a major problem in the community	1	7	3.47	2.13	1	7	4.35	1.91	0.001

in favor of 24-hr containment (30%). Few individuals thought that cats should only be contained during the day or not at all.

Using a 5-point Likert type scale (anchored by 1 = very unimportant and 5 = very important), respondents were also asked to indicate the extent to which they considered it important to confine a cat in each of three containment scenarios: during the day; during the night; or 24-hr containment. Table 2 shows that non-owners consistently placed greater importance on containment than did cat owners. With the exception of general agreement that containment during the night was important, cat owners indicated a degree of ambivalence towards containment during the day or 24-hr containment. A series of Mann-Whitney *U* Tests revealed that, with the exception of beliefs regarding the need for cats to roam, opinions about the importance of cat containment, general feelings towards cats, and beliefs about cats differed significantly between non-owners and owners. In general, non-owners indicated significantly greater support for each cat containment scenario, expressed less positive feelings towards cats, and were more likely to hold negative beliefs about cats.

Choosing as many options as apply, respondents were asked to indicate whether they agreed that cat containment was important for the specified reasons listed, to indicate whether they had observed any of the behaviors listed that wandering cats may engage in, and to indicate whether they were fond of cats (on a binary scale; yes/no). Table 3 shows the number and percentage of respondents (categorized by cat ownership status) who indicated support for the reasons listed. As can be seen, a significantly larger proportion of cat owners considered cat containment important for the purpose of protecting cats from injury than did non-owners (75.4% versus 53.5%; $\chi^2_{(1)}$ = 17.54, *n* = 399, *p* < 0.001). A somewhat higher proportion of non-owners thought that containment was important to protect neighbors from nuisance behavior than did cat owners (58.3% versus 51.6%), although this difference was not significant. Both groups considered cat containment important for the purpose of protecting native wildlife,

Table 3. Frequency of agreement with beliefs about containment, wandering cats, and fondness for cats as a function of cat ownership.

Beliefs		Non-Owners	Cat Owners	p
Containment	To protect them from injury	144 (53.5%)	98 (75.4%)	0.001
	To protect native wildlife	210 (76.9%)	100 (78.1%)	> 0.05
	To protect neighbors from nuisance behavior	158 (58.3%)	65 (51.6%)	> 0.05
	To reduce unwanted breeding	142 (54%)	68 (56.2%)	> 0.05
Wandering Cats	Endanger or kill native wildlife	115 (63.2%)	60 (63.2%)	> 0.05
	Mate	60 (33.9%)	29 (31.5%)	> 0.05
	Fight	118 (65.5%)	69 (73.4%)	> 0.05
	Engage in territorial behavior	101 (57.1%)	62 (67.4%)	> 0.05
Attitudes towards Cats	Fondness	140 (50.0%)	129 (90.8%)	0.001

Table 4. Pearson's correlation coefficients between beliefs and attitudes towards cats and containment importance ratings.

		Containment Importance Ratings for Each Scenario					
		Cat Owner (n = 91–140)			Non-Owner (n = 173–280)		
Beliefs and Attitudes		Day	Night	24 hr	Day	Night	24 hr
Containment Is Important	To protect the cat from injury	−0.01	0.27**	−0.03	0.04	0.12	0.10
	To protect native wildlife	0.15	0.20*	0.15	0.90	0.34**	0.23**
	To protect neighbors from nuisance behavior	0.13	0.11	0.10	0.16*	0.22**	0.21**
	To reduce unwanted breeding	0.04	0.07	0.06	0.10	0.18**	0.12
Wandering Cats	Endanger or kill native wildlife	0.20*	0.10	0.28**	0.12	0.19*	0.21**
	Mate	0.07	−0.11	0.05	0.15*	0.13	0.15
	Fight	−0.04	0.09	0.00	0.17*	0.17*	0.18*
	Engage in territorial behavior	0.04	0.22*	0.12	0.03	0.10	0.09
Attitude towards Cats	Fondness	−0.06	0.01	−0.06	−0.19**	−0.01	−0.12*
	General feelings	−0.15	−0.09	−0.08	−0.31**	−0.07	−0.22**
Beliefs Relating to Cats	Cats pose a serious threat to native wildlife	0.13	0.24**	0.11	0.13*	0.25**	0.22**
	Cats do not need to roam	0.04	0.02	0.03	0.22**	0.07	0.12*
	Many people own too many cats	0.00	0.15	0.07	0.17**	0.04	0.13*
	In general, cats are a major problem in the community	−0.02	0.24**	0.03	0.24**	0.09	0.20**

*p < 0.05, **p < 0.01

Table 5. Resources provided by owners to cats during containment.

Resources	Provided		Not Provided	
	n	%	*n*	%
Food	95	82.6	20	17.4
Bedding	94	81.7	21	18.3
Access to water	89	77.4	26	22.6
Companionship	64	55.7	51	44.3
Litter tray	62	53.9	53	46.1
Toys	58	50.4	57	49.6
Opportunity to exercise	57	50.0	57	50.0
Access to fresh air	57	49.6	58	50.4
Access to sun	53	46.1	62	53.9
Opportunity to engage in normal behaviors	51	44.7	63	55.3
Scratching post	45	39.5	69	60.5
Training	22	19.3	92	80.7

Table 6. Forward Binomial Stepwise Logistic Regression model.

Step	Variable Type	Variables
1	Demographic	Gender
		Age group
		Education
		Relationship status
		Residential location
2	Knowledge	Knowledge regarding cat and dog behavior
3	Cat specific attitudes	Positive cat attributes
		Negative cat attributes
		Independence cat attributes
		Beliefs about cat behavior
		General feeling towards cats
4	Dog specific attitudes	Positive dog attributes
		Negative dog attributes
		Independence dog attributes
		Beliefs about dog behavior
		General feeling towards dogs
5	Containment beliefs	Importance of day containment
		Importance of night containment

whereas fewer respondents thought containment was important to reduce unwanted breeding. No significant differences were observed between groups in relation to the frequency with which they agreed that wandering cats endanger native wildlife, mate, fight, or engage in territorial behavior. Significantly more owners indicated a fondness for cats in comparison with non-owners (98.8% versus 50%; $\chi^2_{(1)}$ = 68.01, *n* = 422, *p* < 0.001). A series of chi-square analyses revealed that there were no significant differences in the

Table 7. Summary of logistic regression analysis predicting containment in cat owners.

	Predictors	B	SE	Wald	p	OR	CI
Day	Beliefs about the importance of daytime containment	1.06	0.21	26.54	0.000	2.88	1.93–4.31
Night	Beliefs about the importance of night containment	0.65	0.21	9.84	0.002	1.92	1.28–2.88

Note: Only variables that achieved significance are presented.

relative frequency with which individuals endorsed a reason for cat containment as a function of their residential location.

Relationships between importance ratings relating to containment during the day, night or 24 hr and a diverse array of beliefs relating to cats wandering at large were examined using Pearson's correlation co-efficients for owner and non-owner groups (Table 4). A high degree of consistency was found in owners and non-owners across beliefs relating to the importance of the three containment scenarios and beliefs regarding the potential threat that cats pose to native wildlife. Conversely, beliefs relating to the importance of containment in non-owners, but not owners, were also related to concerns regarding the potential nuisance that cats may present to the community. In keeping with this, an inverse relationship between general feelings/fondness for cats and beliefs regarding each of the three containment scenarios was observed in non-owners.

Cat owners were asked to indicate their containment behaviors. Eighty percent of cat owners contained their cat to a property during the night, whereas only 41.2% contained their cat to a property during the day. Only 25.7% of cat owners indicated that they had an enclosed yard or cat run. At least 70% of owners residing in each location (urban, suburban, regional city, semi-rural, and rural) indicated that they contained their cat/s at night, with greater likelihood of this behavior observed in respondents residing in urban or suburban locations.

Containment Enrichment

Table 5 shows the resources provided by owners for their contained cats. As can be seen, there is some variation in frequencies across the categories, with essentials such as food and water more likely to be provided than enrichment items, such as toys and companionship.

Predicting Containment Behaviors in Cat Owners

Forward Stepwise Binary Logistic Regression (SLR) was used to identify the demographic, knowledge, belief, and attitudinal factors (relating to companion animal ownership) that predict cat containment behaviors in cat owners (Table 6). Behaviors of interest were whether owners contained a cat to a property during the day or the night, as indexed in binary form (yes/no).

Containment During the Day: As can be seen in Table 7, a significant SLR model was achieved ($\chi^2_{(1)} = 35.51$, $p < 0.001$), with an overall classification accuracy of 73.5% (with 78.8% of respondents who do not, and 66.1% of those who do, contain their cat during the day correctly classified). The only variable that significantly predicted containment behaviors during the day in cat owners was "beliefs regarding the importance of containment."

Containment at Night: Table 7 also shows that a significant SLR model for night containment was achieved ($\chi^2_{(1)} = 10.23$, $p < 0.001$). Using a cut value of 0.65, the model achieved an overall classification accuracy of 80.3% (with 25.9% of those who do not, and 93.6% of those that do, contain their cats at night correctly classified). The only variable to significant predict night containment behaviors in cat owners was "beliefs regarding the importance of containment."

Discussion

The aim of this study was to explore community attitudes and behaviors in relation to cat containment in Australia. The findings revealed a high proportion (80%) of cat owners contain their cat/s to a property at night, whereas only 41.2% contain their cat/s during the day. Mean importance ratings pertaining to cat containment were consistent with these findings, such that containment at night was viewed by owners and non-owners as more important than containment during the day. In general, however, non-owners reported having been disturbed more often by wandering cats, were significantly more in favor of 24-hr containment, and considered it more important compared with cat owners. As expected, owners were significantly more likely to consider containment important for the purpose of protecting cats from injury than were non-owners. However, owners were just as likely as non-owners to endorse containment for the purpose of protecting wildlife. Moreover, this was the most frequent reason given in both groups as to why containment was important, such that importance ratings for confinement were most highly correlated with concerns relating to native wildlife.

These concerns are consistent with past research undertaken in Australia (DSE 1999; Perry 1999; Chaseling 2001) and suggest that education programs pertaining to this issue may have been successful. To date, research that explores public opinion in relation to the imperatives for cat control legislation has been largely confined to Australia (van Heezik 2010); multidisciplinary research is needed to determine whether similar concerns regarding wildlife predation underwrite support for cat containment elsewhere. In addition, the extent of the actual threat that cats pose to native wildlife populations remains uncertain (Lilith et al. 2006). For instance, Barratt (1997) found that native wildlife comprised less than 20% of the species predated on by domestic cats. It is also widely acknowledged that the extent of the threat is moderated by the characteristics of the environment, with native fauna more at risk in pastoral environments, by virtue of their availability.

Thirty percent of Victorian councils have mandated cat confinement legislation in response to the perceived needs of their area; however, owner compliance is difficult to regulate. In this context, it is interesting to note that a significant relationship between concerns relating to the protection of cats from injury and importance ratings of night containment was identified in cat owners. These concerns were not related to daytime or 24-hr containment, which may indicate that owners do not perceive these as important issues during the day. Hence, to encourage containment in regions with 24-hr cat curfew laws in place, further education regarding the potential for harm to occur to cats wandering "at large" during the day may be a useful promotion strategy, particularly in urban and suburban environments.

In general, the importance of containment to non-owners was correlated with concerns relating to the protection of wildlife and community members from harm or nuisance, respectively. Non-owners did not advocate containment for the purpose of protecting cats from injury. Indeed, there was an inverse relationship between fondness for cats in general and the importance of containment, suggesting that non-owners may consider cat containment primarily important for the protection of others. It is interesting that fondness for cats in owners was generally not related to the perceived importance of containment. The only correlation to emerge in this regard revealed a negative association between general feelings for cats and the importance of day containment, suggesting that owners less fond of cats were likely to endorse daytime containment. This suggests that containment practices, particularly during the day, are not yet considered an essential component of responsible animal ownership in owners.

The findings revealed that beliefs relating to the importance of containment predicted engagement in containment behaviors in cat owners. This finding is broadly consistent with the Theory of Planned Behavior, which suggests that attitudes, perceived personal agency, and normative beliefs influence intentions to perform specific behaviors (Fishbein and Ajzen 1975). Given the salience of cat containment issues (such as for the purpose of wildlife protection), it would be interesting to determine the relative influence of social norms on containment behaviors in future research; cross-cultural work of this nature is presently underway. These findings further support the suggestion that owners may benefit from education relating to the importance of containment during the day for the protection of cats, and native wildlife, from harm.

It is likely that information relating to appropriate enrichment strategies would be important in such programs. At present, it appears as though most owners offer access to food, water, and bedding during containment. Notably, however, approximately 20% of cat owners did not report providing these basic necessities to their contained cats. As expected, only 50% of owners offered enrichment opportunities (i.e., toys, scratching post, and companionship) to their contained cats. It is possible that owners do not perceive enrichment as important. However, given that cats are primarily contained at night and are nocturnal animals (and therefore active at night), education relating to these issues would appear worthwhile. In this context, further research that identifies the specific enrichment needs of neutered domestic cats is needed to optimize welfare outcomes.

In summary, the results of this survey indicate the salience of cat containment issues to the general community. Support for containment in non-owners relates largely to the protection of native wildlife from harm and community members from nuisance behaviors. Cat owners believe containment during the night is important as it protects cats from injury. To maximize owner compliance with cat curfew legislation, education programs that highlight what is known about the potential dangers faced by cats wandering at large during the day, in addition to the benefits that may be accrued to cats, native wildlife, and the general community by containment to a suitably enriched property, are needed. These programs should emphasize the welfare requirements of contained cats, including their basic necessities (i.e., access to food, water, and bedding) and enrichment needs (i.e., scratching post, opportunities to engage in "normal" activities); it would be worthwhile monitoring community knowledge and attitudes towards containment issues in response to any such educational campaigns. Given the present day trend for local councils to introduce cat curfew legislation, the question as to whether 24-hr cat containment should be adopted as a nationwide animal management strategy will need to be closely examined. In this context, high quality research that comprehensively documents the advantages and disadvantages of containment to cats, native wildlife, and the community is needed.

Acknowledgements

We gratefully acknowledge the financial support of the Bureau of Animal Welfare, Department of Primary Industries, Victoria and the research assistance of Leila Greenfield.

References

Ajzen, I. and Fishbein, M. 1980. *Understanding Attitudes and Predicting Social Behavior.* Englewood Cliffs, NJ: Prentice Hall.

Australian Bureau of Statistics. 2005a. 6302.0—Average Weekly Earnings, Australia EMBARGO. Census of Population and Housing. <http://www.abs.gov.au/Ausstats/abs@.nsf/> Accessed August 12, 2005.

Australian Bureau of Statistics. 2005b. 6227.0—Education and Work, Australia, May 2005. <http://www.abs.gov.au> Accessed July 25, 2006.

Baldock, C. 1999. Australia's declining household cat population—forecasts, impacts and reasons. A report of an analysis. AusVet Animal Health Services Pty Ltd.

Baldock, F. C. Alexander, L. and More, S. J. 2003. Estimated and predicted changes in the cat population of Australian households from 1979 to 2005. *Australian Veterinary Journal* 81: 289–292.

Barratt, D. G. 1997. Predation by house cats, *Felis catus* (L.), in Canberra, Australia. I. Prey composition and preference. *Wildlife Research* 24: 263–277.

Bernstein, P. L. 2007. The human–cat relationship. In *The Welfare of Cats,* 47–89, ed. I. Rochlitz. Dordrecht, The Netherlands: Springer.

Bradshaw, J. W. S. 1992. *The Behaviour of the Domestic Cat*. Wallingford, Oxon: C. A. B. International.

Calver, M., Thomas, S., Bradley, S. and McCutcheon, H. 2007. Reducing the rate of predation on wildlife by pet cats: The efficacy and practicability of collar-mounted pounce protectors. *Biological Conservation* 137: 341–348.

Chaseling, S. 2001. Pet populations in Australia. Dogs increasing and cats decreasing—why is it so? Urban Animal Management: Proceedings of the National Conference Melbourne, Australia 2001. Australian Veterinary Association, NSW. <http://www.aiam.com.au/resources/files/proceedings/melbourne2001/PUB_Pro01_SusieChasling.pdf> Accessed April 5, 2001.

Coleman, G. J., McGregor, M., Hemsworth, P. H., Boyce, J. and Dowling, S. 2003. The relationship between beliefs, attitudes and observed behaviours of abattoir personnel in the pig industry. *Applied Animal Behaviour Science* 82: 189–200.

Dabritz, H. A. Atwill, E. R., Gardner, I. A., Miller, M. A. and Conrad, P. A. 2006. Outdoor fecal deposition by free-roaming cats and attitudes of cat owners and nonowners toward stray pets, wildlife, and water pollution. *Journal of the American Veterinary Medical Association* 229: 74–81.

Dabritz, H. A. and Conrad, P. A. 2010. Cats and Toxoplasma: Implications for public health. *Zoonoses and Public Health* 57: 34–52.

Department of Sustainability and Environment. 1999. Cats and wildlife—how you can protect both. <http://www.dse.vic.gov.au/dse> Accessed April 29, 2005.

Department of Sustainability and Environment. 2003. Protect your cat. Protect your wildlife. <http://www.nre.vic.gov.au> Accessed March 10, 2004.

Fishbein, M. and Ajzen, I. 1975. *Belief, Attitude, Intention, and Behavior: An Introduction to Theory and Research.* Reading, MA: Addison-Wesley.

Glen, A. S. and Dickman, C. R. 2008. Niche overlap between marsupial and eutherian carnivores: Does competition threaten the endangered spotted-tailed quoll? *Journal of Applied Ecology* 45: 700–707.

Grayson, J., Calver, M. and Styles, I. 2002. Attitudes of suburban Western Australians to proposed cat control legislation. *Australian Veterinary Journal* 80: 536–543.

Jackson, V. 1996. Rethinking approaches to urban animal management: A review and integration of the strategies available. Urban Animal Management: Proceedings of the National Conference, Sydney, Australia 1996. NSW: Australian Veterinary Association. <http://www.aiam.com.au/resources/files/proceedings/sydney1996/PUB_Pro96_VirginiaJackson.pdf> Accessed April 5, 2011.

Jarman, P. and van der Lee, G. 1993. Cats (domestic, stray and feral) and endangered Australian wildlife: A factual review. A report to The Petcare Information and Advisory Service. University of New England, Armidale.

Jones, B. and McGreevy, P. 2007. How much space does an elephant need? The impact of confinement on animal welfare. *Journal of Veterinary Behavior* 2: 185–187.

Jongman, E. C. 2007. Adaptation of domestic cats to confinement. *Journal of Veterinary Behavior* 2: 193–196

Lilith, M., Calver, M., Styles, I. and Garkaklis, M. 2006. Protecting wildlife from predation by owned domestic cats: Application of a precautionary approach to the acceptability of proposed cat regulations. *Austral Ecology* 31: 176–189.

Munro, H. M. C. and Thrusfield, M. V. 2001. "Battered pets": Non-accidental physical injuries found in dogs and cats. *Journal of Small Animal Practice* 42: 279–290.

Nutter, F. B., Levine, J. F. and Stoskopf, M. K. 2004. Reproductive capacity of free-roaming domestic cats and kitten survival rate. *Journal of the American Veterinary Medical Association* 225: 1399–1402.

Perry, G. 1999. Cats – perceptions and misconceptions: Two recent studies about cats and how people see them. Urban Animal Management: Proceedings of the 8th National Conference, Gold Coast, Australia 1999. NSW: Australian Veterinary Association. <http://www.aiam.com.au/resources/files/proceedings/gold-coast1999/PUB_Pro99_GaillePerry.pdf> Accessed April 5, 2011.

Rochlitz, I. 2004. The effects of road traffic accidents on domestic cats and their owners. *Animal Welfare* 13: 51–55.

Rochlitz, I. 2005. A review of the housing requirements of domestic cats (*Felis silvestris catus*) kept in the home. *Applied Animal Behaviour Science* 93: 97–109.

Scriggins, S. and Murray, D. 1997. Cat management for Magnetic Island – a controlled trial. Urban Animal Management: Proceedings of the National Conference, Adelaide, Australia 1997. NSW: Australian Veterinary Association. <http://www.aiam.com.au/resources/files/proceedings/adelaide1997/PUB_Pro97_ShaneScriggins_DickMurray.pdf> Accessed April 5, 2011.

Toukhsati, S. R., Bennett, P. C. and Coleman, G. J. 2007. Behaviors and attitudes towards semi-owned cats. *Anthrozoös* 20: 131–142.

Van de Kuyt, N. 2004. Turning research into reality: how councils can use findings from a survey to help manage pets in the community. Proceedings from the Urban Animal Management National Conference, Adelaide, Australia 2004. NSW: Australian Veterinary Association. <http://www.aiam.com.au/resources/files/proceedings/adelaide2004/PUB_Pro04_VandeKuyt_TurningResearch.pdf> Accessed April 5, 2011.

van Heezik, Y. 2010. Pussyfooting around the issue of cat predation in urban areas. *Oryx* 44: 153–154.

Verbeke, W. 2002. A shift in public opinion. *Pig Progress* 18(2): 25–27.

Verbeke, W. and Vackier, I. 2004. Profile and effects of consumer involvement in fresh meat. *Meat Science* 67(1): 159–168.

ANTHROZOÖS   VOLUME 25, ISSUE 1   REPRINTS AVAILABLE   PHOTOCOPYING   © ISAZ 2012
PP. 75–91   DIRECTLY FROM   PERMITTED   PRINTED IN THE UK
THE PUBLISHERS   BY LICENSE ONLY

Perceptions of Village Dogs by Villagers and Tourists in the Coastal Region of Rural Oaxaca, Mexico

Eliza Ruiz-Izaguirre and Catharina Helena Antonia Maria Eilers

Animal Production Systems Group, Department of Animal Sciences, Wageningen University, The Netherlands

Address for correspondence:
Eliza Ruiz Izaguirre,
Animal Production Systems Group,
PO Box 338,
6700 AH Wageningen,
The Netherlands.
E-mail:
eliza.ruizizaguirre@gmail.com

ABSTRACT The objective of this study was to gain an understanding of the village dog-keeping system, and of perceptions of dog-related problems by villagers and tourists, in the coastal region of Oaxaca, Mexico. We conducted a survey of the inhabitants of three villages (Mazunte, Puerto Angel, and Río Seco), whose main economic activities were tourism, fishing, and farming ($n = 99$), and a survey of tourists ($n = 151$). Dogs were the most commonly kept animals in all the villages. Cultural and economic aspects were reflected in dog-keeping practices. All dog owners allowed their dog(s) to roam free in the farming village (Río Seco), but not in the tourist villages (Mazunte and Puerto Angel). Significantly more dog owners in the tourist village of Mazunte mentioned companionship as a reason for keeping dogs than those in the farming village. All villagers perceived as a problem that there were too many dogs. The mean number of dogs per household was 1.8, and there were significantly more male dogs in the farming village than in the tourist villages. Efforts to control the dog population in the rural coastal region are aimed at rabies prevention or wildlife protection, whereas this study revealed that these issues were far less often mentioned by local people as other dog-related problems. Significantly more villagers in the tourist villages perceived there to be dog-welfare problems than those in the farming village. Significantly more North American and European tourists were concerned about dog welfare than Mexican tourists. Despite significant differences in dog-keeping between the tourist and farming villages, opinions of villagers in regard to dog breeding and methods of dog population control were similar. Villagers agreed on dog sterilization to control the dog population, but also considered that female dogs should breed at least once in their lifetime. Those living in tourist villages could benefit from improving dog welfare and implementing strategies to lessen the problems dogs cause tourists.

Anthrozoös   DOI: 10.2752/175303712X13240472427555

Keywords: dog, dog-keeping, dog welfare, Mexico

 Dogs that are free to roam outside household premises are commonly known as "village dogs" (Coppinger and Coppinger 2001; Boitani, Ciucci and Ortolani 2007; Ortolani, Vernooij and Coppinger 2009), and this could be the most common dog category in developing countries (Ortolani, Vernooij and Coppinger 2009). In rural areas of Mexico, for example, most households (60–85%) own dogs (Orihuela and Solano 1995; Ortega-Pacheco et al. 2007), which is different from other countries, where people do not acknowledge ownership of village dogs (Ortolani, Vernooij and Coppinger 2009). Village dogs in the coastal region of rural Oaxaca, Mexico roam the beaches and streets, just as in other parts of Mexico (Orihuela and Solano 1995; Ortega-Pacheco et al. 2007).

Tourism is an important economic activity for seaside villages of the coastal region, and it has brought an influx of foreigners who may have different perceptions of dogs (Plumridge and Fielding 2003). It is known locally that tourists interact with village dogs by feeding them and sometimes by adopting them. This coastal region of rural Oaxaca, furthermore, has gained attention from foreign veterinarians, who perform an annual dog sterilization campaign there (Borgal 2001).

Most studies regarding village dogs in developing countries have focused on rabies and other zoonoses (Slater 2001), whereas other dog-related problems that are also relevant, for example, overpopulation and free-roaming dogs, have received less attention. There are four main concerns regarding dogs in the coastal region of Oaxaca: overpopulation, welfare, free-roaming, and threat to wildlife. Dog overpopulation has been reported also in other parts of Mexico (Orihuela and Solano 1995; Ortega-Pacheco et al. 2007) and, in general, in areas of developing countries (Butler and Bingham 2000; Kitala et al. 2001; Fraser 2008). Dog welfare is regarded as poor not only in coastal tourist sites in the Caribbean (Grennan and Fielding 2008), but also in developing countries (Fraser 2008). Free-roaming dogs could give tourists a bad impression of the community (Plumridge and Fielding 2003; Alie et al. 2007), and this may affect the local economy (Plumridge and Fielding 2003). Dogs may pose a threat to wildlife in nature-protected areas (Slater 2001); in the coastal region of Oaxaca, for example, dogs are known to feed on sea turtle nests.

In the search for solutions to dog-related problems, opinions of stakeholders are rarely considered, unlike for some animal species, for example, dingoes in Australia (Burns 2003) and iguanas in Central America (Eilers et al. 2001). Stakeholders are those individuals who can affect a "system," in this case a "dog-keeping system." A system is a construct used to understand complex reality in a particular context (Udo and Cornelissen 1998). A systems approach, therefore, takes into account how stakeholders, animals, and the environment interrelate. According to a systems approach, it is important to understand first the system before trying to change it (Udo and Cornelissen 1998). Often, solutions are designed with top-down approaches, not taking into account views of stakeholders who will be affected and who will have influence in the success or failure of a solution. For this study, we considered two groups of stakeholders: villagers and tourists. The objective of this study was to gain further understanding of the dog-keeping systems in villages, and of perceptions of dog-related problems by villagers and tourists in the rural coastal region of Oaxaca, Mexico. We studied dog-keeping systems and the opinions of villagers in three different villages: one farming village and two tourist villages. We hypothesized that perceptions of village dogs by tourists would influence the perceptions of dogs by villagers— for example, making them more aware of dog-welfare problems.

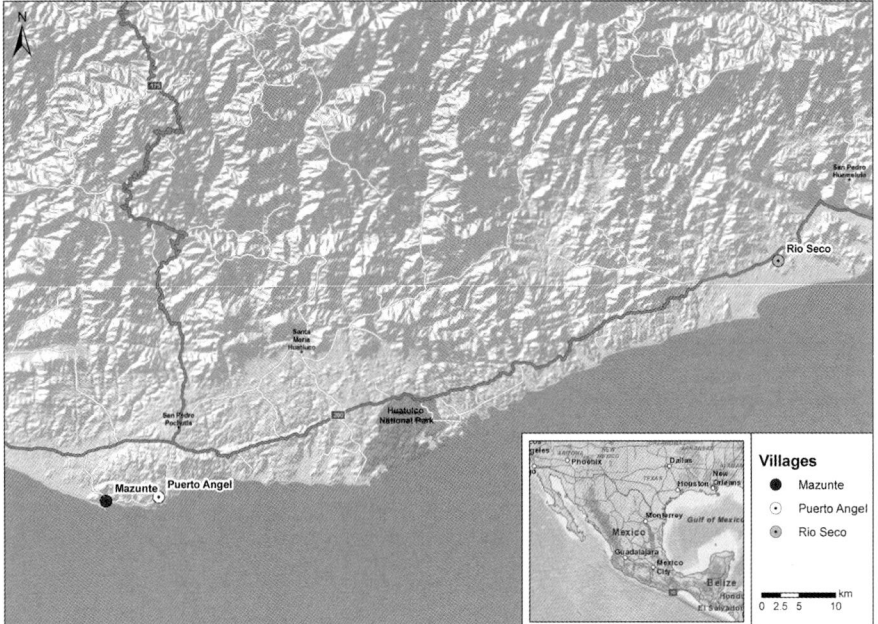

Figure 1. Villages surveyed in the Coastal Region of Oaxaca, Mexico.

Methods
Study Sites
The coastal region of the State of Oaxaca is located on the South Pacific Coast of Mexico. This region is known for its sea turtle nesting sanctuaries: La Escobilla and Morro Ayuta (SEMARNAT and CONANP 2006), and for its tourist resorts: Bahías de Huatulco and Puerto Escondido (Foucat 2002). Tourists visiting Bahías de Huatulco often visit the neighboring villages of Ventanilla, Mazunte, and Puerto Angel (Foucat 2002). Bahías de Huatulco generated 48% of the total tourist income for Oaxaca in 2006, and Ventanilla-Puerto Angel, known as the rural eco-tourist area, generated 3% (Boletín Estadístico 2006).

This study was conducted in January and February 2006. The Mexican Turtle Center (Centro Mexicano de la Tortuga: CMT) was concerned about dog-related problems, for example, dog overpopulation and predation of sea turtle (*Lepidochelys olivacea*) nests in rural villages of the coastal region of Oaxaca. To determine the influence of tourists on village dog-keeping systems, we selected two rural seashore villages with tourists—Mazunte and Puerto Angel—and one rural inland village without tourists—Río Seco (Figure 1). The villages are representative of rural communities with fewer than 2,500 inhabitants, and were known by the CMT to have problems with village dogs.

The main economic activities of the villages are tourism (Mazunte and Puerto Angel), fishing (Puerto Angel), and farming (Río Seco). The ethnic composition is mostly indigenous (Chontales) in Río Seco and mostly mestizo in Puerto Angel and Mazunte, the latter with growing numbers of European and North American expatriates. Río Seco is the most rural of the three villages, and Puerto Angel the least. According to the latest census (2005), Mazunte had 702 inhabitants and 153 houses, Puerto Angel had 2,440 inhabitants and 153 houses, and Río Seco had 647 inhabitants and 186 houses (INEGI 2005).

Table 1. Summary of the questions asked (and possible answers) during the surveys of the villagers.

Background of Respondent

Age (14–20/21–30/31–40/41–50/more than 50 years old)

Gender (female/male)

Nationality

Number of years residing in the village

Education level (primary/secondary/high school/university)

Do you own land for farming? (yes/no)

Is your salary enough to maintain your family? (yes/no)

Do you own animals? (yes/no)

Animal species owned (dogs, cats, birds, poultry, cattle, sheep/goats, horses)

    If you own animals, which animal species is the most important for the household?

Problems and Opinions Regarding Village Dogs

Which is the most important problem in the village? (open question)

Do you consider that there are problems in regard to village dogs? (yes/no)

Which problems do you experience with village dogs? (open question)

Have you ever been bitten by a dog? (yes/no)

Have you lately been chased by a dog or a group of dogs? (yes/no)

Have you ever owned a dog? (yes/no)

    If yes, what was the cause of death or disappearance of your most recent previous dog? (open question)

Do visiting dogs come into your family premises? (yes/no)

Do you feed visiting dogs? (yes/no)

Opinions

Do you agree that dogs should be left free to roam? (yes/no/do not know)

Do you agree that female dogs should be sterilized? (yes/no/do not know)

Do you agree that male dogs should be sterilized? (yes/no/do not know)

Would you be willing to pay for a sterilization surgery? (yes/no/do not know)

    If yes, how much? (in pesos)

Do you agree on poisoning as a dog population control method? (yes/no/do not know)

Would you agree on euthanizing a sick dog with a lethal injection? (yes/no/do not know)

Additional Questions for Dog Owners

Number of male dogs owned

Age of each male dog (< 1/1–3/4–6/> 6 years old)

Number of female dogs owned

Age of each female dog (< 1/1–3/4–6/> 6 years old)

What breeds do you have? (local village dog/ resembling purebred or purebred/ both)

How did you obtain your dog(s)? (gift/bought/found/from own litter)

Why do you keep a dog? (guarding/protection, companionship, state other functions)

How often do you feed your dog(s)? (daily/less than daily)

What does your dog(s) eat? (tortillas, family leftovers, commercial dog food, what the dog scavenges)

Do you have a water tray for your dog (s)? (yes/no)

How often do you replenish the water tray? (daily/every other day/less than every other day)

Do you let your dog(s) roam free? (yes/no)

Have you ever given veterinary treatment your dog(s)? (yes/no)

Do you bathe your dog(s)? (yes/no)

Are your dog(s) rabies vaccinated? (yes/no) (yes means all dogs in the case of multiple dogs)

How many of your dog(s) are sterilized?

Who sterilized your dog(s)? (local vet/ foreign vet campaign)

Río Seco is located 6 km from Morro Ayuta, a sea turtle nesting beach with more than 100,000 nests per year (CONANP 2007); the species status is "vulnerable" (IUCN 2010). Mazunte is located 25 km from La Escobilla, a protected federal beach that holds more than 500,000 nests per year (CONANP 2007). Since 2001, a group from the Massachusetts Veterinary Medical Association, with logistic support from the CMT, have held an annual dog sterilization campaign in Mazunte and Río Seco (personal communication, Richard Rodgers).

Questionnaire Design and Procedure

We used a two-step method to interview our stakeholders: key stakeholder semi-structured interviews and villager and tourist surveys. The objective of the first step was to identify dog-related problems in the area and to develop the questionnaires for the villager and tourist surveys. Key stakeholders were individuals knowledgeable about the dog-keeping practices in the rural system and who considered that dog-related problems should be tackled. We interviewed key stakeholders including workers of the CMT, biologists, local authorities, and veterinarians working in this area.

The objective of the second step was to interview villagers in Mazunte, Puerto Angel and Río Seco, and tourists. We interviewed 99 villagers about the village dogs and keeping dogs. The structured interview consisted of 83 closed-ended and four open-ended questions for dog owners, and 33 closed-ended questions and four open-ended questions for non-dog owners, and lasted from 15 to 45 minutes. The interview covered aspects of village dog-keeping practices and opinions of villagers regarding dog-related problems (Table 1). The interview was initially tested on 10 villagers. Villagers to be interviewed were selected by dividing each village into four areas with the help of a map or, when a map was not available, local authorities. At least seven villagers were interviewed in each area. Two researchers approached every third household and asked the inhabitants to participate. We interviewed 37 villagers in Mazunte, 30 in Puerto Angel, and 32 in Río Seco.

We also surveyed tourists about dog-related problems on the beaches they visited and their interactions with village dogs (Table 2). A sign inviting tourists to participate in the survey was placed in the lobby of the CMT for six weeks in January and February 2006. The survey consisted of 11 closed-ended questions and one open-ended question. In total, 151 questionnaires were completed and analyzed. The complete villager and tourist questionnaires are available from the authors.

Table 2. Summary of the questions (and possible answers) asked of the tourists.

Gender (female/male)
Age (in years)
Nationality
For how long have you been in the coastal region of Oaxaca? (1–7 days/8–15 days/16–30 days/> 30 days)
Places visited (Bahías de Huatulco, Puerto Escondido, Mazunte, Puerto Angel, other)
Do you consider that there are problems related to dogs in the places you have visited? (yes/no)
If yes, which dog-related problems? (select from a list, for example, dogs barking at night, threat to wildlife, bitten by a dog)
Do you consider that something has to be done to control the dog population in this region? (yes/no)
If yes, what can be done? (open question)
Have you fed any dogs during your stay in this coastal region? (daily/sometimes/never)

Analysis

The software package R (R Development Core Team 2010) was used for statistical analysis of the results. Frequencies and percentages of answers on the questionnaires were obtained to characterize the dog-keeping system and to quantify dog-related problems. Villages, dog-keeping systems, and the origin of tourists were analyzed for differences using the chi-square test (Siegel and Castellan 1998).

Results

Villagers

Almost all villagers were Mexican, except for an Italian and a North American who had lived in Mazunte for more than five years. We did not count the number of people who refused to be interviewed, but this was minimal (less than 10%), and mainly occurred in Puerto Angel and Río Seco. Some villagers in Puerto Angel were too busy and some in Río Seco did not feel comfortable talking to strangers. There was no significant difference in the distribution of in-terviewees' ages among the villages (Table 3). We interviewed more women ($n = 65$) than men ($n = 34$), with no significant difference in distribution of gender among villages (Table 3).

In the tourist village Mazunte and the farming village Río Seco, more villagers owned land for farming than in the tourist village Puerto Angel, where fishing was the (other) main economic activity ($\chi^2 = 24.3$, $n = 94$, $df = 2$, $p < 0.001$) (Table 3). With regard to household economy, fewer villagers in Puerto Angel and Río Seco considered family income sufficient than in Mazunte ($\chi^2 = 10.6$, $n = 94$, $df = 2$, $p < 0.01$). Approximately one-third of villagers had completed high school or higher education, with no significant difference in distribution of education level among villages (Table 3).

Tourists

In regard to origin of tourists, 67 were Mexican (44%), 46 North American (United States and Canada) (31%), and 38 European (25%). The mean age of tourists was 33 years ($SD = 13$), ranging from 13 to 69 years ($n = 143$), and there were 90 women (61%) and 57 men (39%). Most tourists ($n = 122$, 81%) had visited Mazunte, but fewer had visited Puerto Angel ($n = 65$, 43%). More than half of the tourists ($n = 82$, 58%) had been in the area for less than one week.

Dog-Keeping Systems

Dogs were the most commonly owned animal species in the three villages, with no significant differences in distribution of species among villages (Table 4). There were, however, differences among villages in the keeping of farm animals, with higher percentages of poultry, horses, pigs, and cattle in Río Seco, reflecting the economic activities of the villages. Villagers were asked which of their animals were most important for the household. Importance could be in relation to utilitarian or affection aspects. Dogs were most important for 22% of villagers, with no significant difference among villages. Horses and poultry were also mentioned as most important, mainly in the farming village. Other animal species were rarely mentioned.

Dog Owners and Their Dogs

Most dog owners ($n = 50$, 78%) owned local village dogs of no specific breed and had acquired their dogs as gifts ($n = 50$, 82%). In the farming village Río Seco, all dog owners ($n = 24$, 100%) allowed their dogs to roam free, but not in Mazunte ($n = 15$, 71%) or Puerto Angel ($n = 16$, 84%). Dog owners gave more than one reason for keeping dogs (Table 5), but almost

Table 3. Villagers' background characteristics.

Characteristics	Level	Mazunte n (%)	Puerto Angel n (%)	Río Seco n (%)
Gender	Female	27 (73)	16 (53)	22 (69)
	Male	10 (27)	14 (47)	10 (31)
Age	14–30 years	15 (41)	9 (30)	11 (34)
	31–50 years	13 (35)	11 (37)	10 (32)
	> 50 years	9 (24)	10 (33)	11 (34)
Owns land for farming***	Yes	18 (51)	3 (10)	22 (73)
	No	17 (49)	23 (90)	8 (27)
Considers income sufficient**	Yes	20 (57)	7 (23)	7 (24)
	No	15 (43)	23 (77)	22 (76)
Education	None or incomplete primary	12 (34)	5 (17)	6 (19)
	Primary	9 (26)	9 (31)	5 (16)
	Secondary	4 (11)	4 (14)	9 (29)
	High school or above	10 (29)	11 (38)	11 (36)

**Different among villages at $p < 0.01$. ***Different among villages at $p < 0.001$.

Table 4. Domestic animals kept by the villagers (%).

Animal Kept	Mazunte n = 37	Puerto Angel n = 32	Río Seco n = 30
Dogs	62	59	78
Poultry*	57	30	72
Birds	35	23	16
Cats	27	23	34
Horses*	10	0	56
Pigs*	8	0	47
Cattle*	0	3	22
Small ruminants	6	0	22

*Different among villages at $p < 0.05$.

Table 5. Reasons for dog-owning villagers to keep dogs (%).

Reason	Mazunte n = 23	Puerto Angel n = 19	Río Seco n = 25	Total n = 67
Guarding/protection	100	95	100	98
Companionship*	78	58	36	57
Playmates for children	45	42	28	38
Protection of backyard animals*	36	10	36	27
Herding cattle or small ruminants*	4	0	28	13
Pest deterrents	36	26	16	26
Work companions	78	52	72	67

*Different among villages at $p < 0.05$.

all mentioned guarding/for protection. Possibly due to the influence of tourists, in Mazunte, more dog owners ($n = 18$) mentioned companionship than owners in the farming village Río Seco ($n = 9$) ($\chi^2 = 7.1$, $df = 1$, $n = 48$, $p < 0.01$). Other reasons for keeping dogs were: play-mates for children, protection of backyard animals (mainly in Mazunte and Río Seco), herding (mainly in Río Seco), and as pest deterrents. Villagers also often mentioned that dogs came along to the fields or followed fishermen to the shore and waited for them until they returned (Table 5, "Work companions").

Feeding of Dogs

Almost all dog owners (98% of 65 replies) fed their dogs daily. All (66 replies) had a water tray for their dog and most owners (86% of 60 replies) replenished the tray every day. In the farming village Río Seco, all dog owners ($n = 25$) fed their dogs maize tortillas with family leftovers, whereas 32% ($n = 7$) of owners in Mazunte and 13% ($n = 2$) in Puerto Angel fed their dogs commercial dog food, exclusively or in addition to leftovers. More than half of villagers (55% of 95 replies) had regular visits by dogs that did not belong to the household ("visiting dogs"), with no significant difference in the distribution of these dogs among villages (Table 8), and 21% of villagers (95 replies) also fed visiting dogs. Non-dog owners ($n = 25$, 83%) were more likely to have visiting dogs than dog owners ($n = 27$, 41%) ($\chi^2 = 12.8$, $df = 1$, $n = 95$, $p < 0.001$), and non-dog owners ($n = 13$, 43%) were also more likely to feed visiting dogs than dog owners ($n = 7$, 11%) ($\chi^2 = 11.2$, $df = 1$, $n = 95$, $p < 0.001$).

Dog Health Care

In the tourist villages Mazunte ($n = 15$, 65%) and Puerto Angel ($n = 10$, 53%), more dog owners gave veterinary treatments to their dogs than owners in the farming village Río Seco ($n = 4$, 17%) ($\chi^2 = 11.3$, $df = 2$, $n = 65$, $p < 0.01$), possibly due to Río Seco not having veterinarians nearby. Veterinary treatments included preventive treatments such as deworming and vaccinations other than rabies. Dogs in Mexico are vaccinated against rabies at no cost during the yearly national rabies campaign (SSA 2001). Possibly due to better vaccination coverage, in Puerto Angel, more dog owners ($n = 16$, 84%) had all their dogs vaccinated against rabies than owners in the farming village Río Seco ($n = 9$, 43%) ($\chi^2 = 5.6$, $df = 1$, $n = 40$, $p < 0.05$). In Mazunte, more dog owners ($n = 19$, 95%) bathed their dogs than owners in Río Seco ($n = 15$, 63%) ($\chi^2 = 4.8$, $df = 1$, $n = 44$, $p < 0.05$).

Causes of Dog Deaths

Most villagers ($n = 81$, 83%) had kept a dog at some point in their lives, with no significant difference in the distribution of dog-keeping among villages. Causes of death or disappearance of the most recent previous dog were: poison (32%), disease (19%), old age (17%), hit by a car (9%), given away (8%), lost (4%), or "other causes" (11%), with no significant difference in the distribution of causes among villages.

Village Dog Population Demographics

We estimated the village dog populations from 121 dogs owned by 67 dog owners (Table 6). The mean number of dogs per household was 1.8. In the farming village Río Seco, there were more male dogs ($n = 38$, 84%) than in the tourist villages Puerto Angel ($n = 21$, 60%) and Mazunte ($n = 21$, 51%) ($\chi^2 = 11.4$, $df = 2$, $n = 121$, $p < 0.01$). This was reflected in an unequal male:female ratio for Puerto Angel and Río Seco (Table 6). In Río Seco, reasons given by villagers to cull newborn female pups were: preference for male dogs as work companions and dislike of "breeding nuisance"—having several males roaming around the household when a

Table 6. Estimated dog population demographics in the three villages.

Demographics	Mazunte	Puerto Angel	Río Seco
Mean no. of dogs/ dog-owning household	1.6	1.8	1.9
Dog male:female ratio**	1:1	1.5:1	5.4:1
Total number of dogs[a]	152	668	276
Human:dog ratio[b]	4:1	4:1	2:1

**Different among villages at $p < 0.01$.

[a]Total number of dogs was calculated by multiplying the mean number of dogs per household by the estimated number of households owning dogs (number of households in 2005 by % of households with dogs in the survey) in the village.

[b]The human:dog ratio was calculated by dividing the total village population by the estimated number of dogs (see [a]).

Table 7. Villagers' opinions ($n = 99$) on dog breeding and other issues (%).

Do You Agree?		Yes	No	Do Not Know
With sterilization of:	Female dogs	98	1	1
	Male dogs	74	21	5
	Specific breeds	59	24	17
That female dogs should breed ($n = 97$)		61 (50)[a]	37	2
That dogs should be free to roam		17	82	1
With poisoning as a method of dog population control		17	81	2
With euthanasia of sick dogs		81	17	2

[a]Villagers considered breeding necessary at least once in the dog's lifetime.

female dog is in heat (see Table 8). In total, few dogs (19% of males, 12% of females) were sterilized, most at no cost during the dog sterilization campaign.

The distribution of ages of the dogs was: 25% under 1 year of age, 40% between 1 and 3 years, 22% between 4 and 6 years, and 13% over 6 years ($n = 118$), with no significant difference in distribution of ages among villages. Most dogs (80%) over 6 years of age were males.

Opinions of Villagers on the Dog-Keeping System

Villagers gave their opinion about various issues regarding dog breeding and methods to control the dog population (Table 7). Opinions of villagers did not differ significantly between dog owners and non-dog owners, or among villages. Most villagers (98%) agreed on sterilization of female dogs, but to a lesser degree on sterilization of male dogs (74%) and of dogs of both sexes of a specific breed (59%) (Table 7). Villagers who disagreed with sterilizing males mentioned one or more reasons, including that guarding behavior will diminish (38%), dog will get lazy (19%), sterilization will be painful (14%), dog will lose masculinity (4%), and sterilization is unnatural (4%).

In regard to female dogs, 61% of villagers agreed they should be allowed to breed, and about half agreed that it should occur at least once in the dog's lifetime. Some villagers explained that "female dogs deserve the opportunity to experience being a mother." Most villagers ($n = 87$, 88%) mentioned willingness to sterilize their dog if it was offered at low cost. Villagers mentioned being able to pay about 20 to 40 pesos (1 Mexican peso = 0.069 EUR, average exchange rate 2006), which was the price of a boar castration. Local veterinarians charged between 300 (male) and 1000 pesos (female) for the surgical sterilization of a dog.

Table 8. Dog-related problems according to villagers and tourists, and respondents' interactions with village dogs (%).

	Villagers				Tourists			
	Mazunte	Puerto Angel	Río Seco	Total	Mexican	European	North American	Total
Problems	$n = 37$	$n = 32$	$n = 30$	$n = 99$	$n = 67$	$n = 38$	$n = 46$	$n = 151$
Too many dogs	46	60	41	48	25	45	37	34
Aggressive dogs	38	33	28	33	–	–	–	–
Dog welfare	40**	40**	9**	30	33***	58***	67***	50
Dog feces	30	30	25	28	43	45	48	45
Dogs spill garbage	35	33	16	28	–	–	–	–
Dogs steal food	32*	7*	34*	25	12	5	9	9
Dogs beg for food	–	–	–	–	27	32	33	30
Breeding nuisance	27	23	22	24	16	5	15	13
Barking at night	19	10	16	15	12***	13***	41***	21
Zoonoses	24	7	9	14	27	34	37	32
Threat to wildlife	0	0	3	3	15**	8**	37**	20
Bad image	19	10	0	10	–	–	–	–
Dog poisoning	11	3	6	7	–	–	–	–
Dogs kill poultry	3	0	19	7	–	–	–	–
Respondents Interactions with Village Dogs								
Have visiting dogs[a]	51	70	37	55	–	–	–	–
Feed (visiting) dogs[b]	9*	40*	17*	20	42	47	31	40
Chased by a dog	8	0	9	6	9	6	7	8
Bitten by a dog[c]	35	47	25	36	3	0	7	3

*Different among villages at $p < 0.05$.

**Different among villages or origins of tourists at $p < 0.01$.

***Different among villages or origins of tourists at $p < 0.001$.

[a]Total n for villagers = 95.

[b]Total n for villagers = 95, total n for tourists = 145.

[c]For villagers (total $n = 96$), the question referred to whether they had been bitten by a dog during their lifetime, whereas for tourists (total $n = 149$), the question referred to being bitten during their stay in the coastal region of Oaxaca.

Most villagers (82%) did not agree with allowing dogs to roam free. Those who agreed mentioned that it was natural for a dog to live this way, and that chained dogs became aggressive. Villagers were asked about two methods of dog culling: poisoning to control the dog population, and euthanasia for sick dogs (with lethal injection). Most villagers (81%) were in favor of euthanasia, whereas a few ($n = 17$) were in favor of poisoning. Dogs that spill garbage, steal food, and kill poultry (see Table 8) were described by villagers as "destructive dogs" (our translation from *dañeros*). Villagers in favor of poisoning mentioned being extremely annoyed by "destructive dogs." Villagers who disagreed with poisoning were annoyed that baits were eaten by dogs that were owned and well cared for, and they were afraid that baits could be eaten by small children.

Damage to Sea Turtle Nests

In Río Seco, villagers reported the presence of *perros salvajes* (feral dogs), described as dogs that avoid humans and live independently on the beach Morro Ayuta, which is a sea turtle nesting site. Villagers mentioned that feral dogs dig out and eat sea turtle eggs, and this was confirmed by one of the authors (E. R.).

Perceptions of Dog-Related Problems by Villagers and Tourists

Villagers were asked about the main village problems, to place dog-related problems in a wider socio-economic context. The main village problems included drug addiction and drug trafficking (Mazunte), bad drainage systems (Puerto Angel), and lack of jobs (Río Seco). None of the villagers considered dog-related problems as major, but when asked if there were dog-related problems, most villagers answered "Yes" (Mazunte $n = 31$, 86%; Puerto Angel $n = 29$, 96%, and Río Seco $n = 23$, 74%), with no significant difference in the presence of dog-related problems among villages. Perceptions of villagers and tourists, and respondents' interactions with village dogs, are in Table 8. Two main dog-related problems in all villages were that there were too many dogs ($n = 48$) and that there were aggressive dogs ($n = 33$). Too many dogs or overpopulation was also perceived by one-third of tourists. In regard to experience with aggressive dogs, a few villagers were chased by dogs ($n = 6$), and more than one-third of villagers ($n = 35$, of 96 replies) had been bitten by a dog during their lifetimes. A few tourists ($n = 12$) also reported that dogs had chased them, and five tourists (of 149 replies) had been bitten by a dog during their stay.

With regard to dog-welfare problems, we refer to dogs with a visible disease or who are very thin. Dog-welfare problems were reported by villagers and tourists, with differences among villages and among origin of tourists. In the tourist villages, more villagers (Mazunte $n = 15$, Puerto Angel $n = 12$) perceived dog-welfare problems than villagers from Río Seco ($n = 3$) ($\chi^2 = 9.8$, $df = 2$, $n = 99$, $p < 0.01$). More North American ($n = 31$) and European tourists ($n = 22$) perceived dog-welfare problems than Mexican tourists ($n = 22$) ($\chi^2 = 14.4$, $df = 2$, $n = 151$, $p < 0.001$). One-third of villagers were concerned about feces on streets and beaches, whereas almost half of tourists were concerned.

More non-dog owners ($n = 9$, 28%) were disturbed by barking at night than dog owners ($n = 6$, 9%) ($\chi^2 = 4.8$, $n = 99$, $df = 1$, $p < 0.05$). More North Americans ($n = 19$) were disturbed by barking than Europeans ($n = 5$) or Mexican tourists ($n = 8$) ($\chi^2 = 16.0$, $n = 151$, $df = 2$, $p < 0.001$). One-third of tourists ($n = 48$) were concerned about the risk of acquiring zoonotic diseases from the dogs, but zoonoses were not considered a problem by most villagers ($n = 14$). A few villagers in Mazunte ($n = 7$) and Puerto Angel ($n = 3$) mentioned that free-roaming dogs show the community in a bad light to tourists.

One-third of tourists ($n = 45$) found it annoying to see dogs beg for food in restaurants. More than one-third of tourists ($n = 58$), nonetheless, gave food to village dogs during their visit ("daily" or "sometimes"). Possibly because there were plenty of fish leftovers, more villagers in Puerto Angel ($n = 12$) fed visiting dogs than villagers in Mazunte ($n = 3$) ($\chi^2 = 7.3$, $df = 1$, $n = 65$, $p < 0.01$), and fewer villagers in Puerto Angel were concerned with dogs stealing food ($n = 2$) than villagers in Mazunte ($n = 12$) and Río Seco ($n = 11$) ($\chi^2 = 7.9$, $df = 2$, $n = 99$, $p < 0.05$).

A few villagers, especially in Mazunte, were concerned about dogs being poisoned en masse. More North Americans ($n = 17$) were concerned about dogs being a threat to wildlife than Mexicans ($n = 10$) or Europeans ($n = 3$) ($\chi^2 = 12.9$, $df = 2$, $n = 151$, $p < 0.01$). Only three

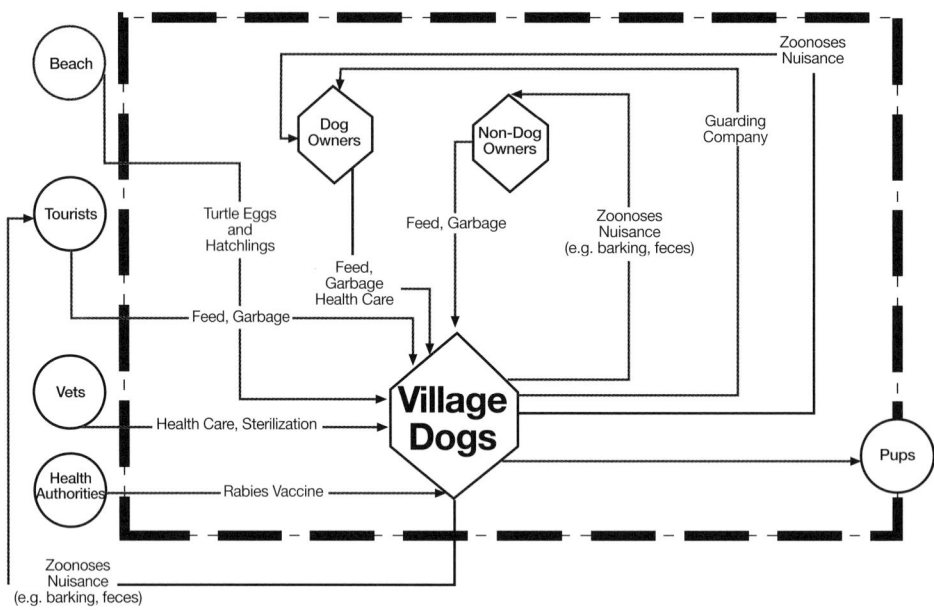

Figure 2. Village dog-keeping-system in rural Oaxaca, Mexico.

villagers in Río Seco were specifically concerned that village dogs ate turtle eggs and hatchlings.

Tourists were asked if they considered it necessary to control the village dog population and, if so, to mention possible control methods. Most ($n = 121$, 83%) considered control of the dog population necessary, with no significant difference in opinion by origin of tourists ($n = 146$). Tourists ($n = 96$, 67%) suggested control methods, which were (in order of frequency): sterilize the dog, make owners responsible, build animal shelters, euthanize sick dogs, prohibit free-roaming, and allow only one or two dogs per household.

Figure 2 summarizes the dog-keeping system of the coastal villages studied. Village dogs get food from multiple sources, such as garbage and are given food from tourists and villagers (dog owners and non-dog owners), as well as from sea turtle nests. Village dogs get health care from veterinarians, Mexican health authorities, and their owners. Despite the various functions of village dogs, such as for protection and companionship, these animals cause various problems for villagers and tourists, such as defecating on the street and barking. Additionally, dogs may transmit zoonotic diseases to villagers and tourists, even though villagers do not acknowledge this as a problem.

Discussion

Village Dog Population Demographics

The dog population demographics in this study are similar to those found in some other dog population studies: sex bias for males over females and low life expectancy (Orihuela and Solano 1995; Butler and Bingham 2000; Kitala et al. 2001; Ortega-Pacheco et al. 2007). The male:female ratio in Río Seco is higher than in other studies, but similar to what was found in rural areas of Chile (Acosta-Jamett et al. 2010). In our study, this is explained by the preference for male dogs and the culling of female pups. This finding supports the hypothesis that the sex bias in dogs may be anthropogenic in nature (Macpherson, Meslin and Wandeler 2000). The number of dogs per household (ranging from 1.6 to 1.9) and the human:dog ratio (ranging from 2:1 to 4:1) are similar to those found for rural villages in Yucatán, Mexico (Ortega-Pacheco et al. 2007).

Although in the tourist villages dogs got better health care (more visits to a veterinarian, vaccinations, and bathing) than in the farming village, there were very few dogs older than 6 years in all the villages, which indicates a rapid population turnover. A rapid population turnover is characteristic of village dogs with high fecundity and low survivorship (Kitala et al. 2001). It is possible that in all three villages, dogs are exposed to the risks of being poisoned or being hit by a car.

Free-Roaming Dogs

Village dogs have been present in Mexico for at least 4,000 years before colonization by the Spanish (Valadez-Azúa and Mestre-Arrioja 1999) and were most likely roaming free. Before Spanish colonization, the identity of a *perro callejero* (stray dog) did not exist or was not seen as disagreeable and giving a bad image (Valadez-Azúa and Mestre-Arrioja 1999). This agrees with what we found in the (indigenous) farming village Río Seco, where all dogs roamed free and nobody was concerned with dogs projecting a bad image. We agree with Poss and Bader (2007), therefore, that the culture of Latin-American people may be an important component in allowing dogs to roam free, and it would be enlightening to study this relation between dogs and culture in more detail.

We believe that dog-keeping practices and perceptions in regard to free-roaming dogs are also influenced by current tourist development. In the tourist villages, unlike in the farming village, not all owners allowed their dogs to roam free, and some villagers were concerned about dogs giving the village a bad image. Allowing dogs to roam free may have advantages over keeping dogs enclosed because it reduces the work, management, and costs of keeping dogs; for example, both dog owners and non-dog owners were involved in feeding visiting dogs. Allowing dogs to roam free, however, also has disadvantages for villagers: villagers complained about aggressive dogs and various other dog problems. Although a few villagers and tourists were chased and bitten by dogs, the problem of aggressive dogs seems to be of a lesser degree than was found in a Latino community in Texas, where most respondents (81%, *n* = 165) answered that free-roaming dogs prevented them from walking outside (Poss and Bader 2007). In New Providence, The Bahamas, dog barking at night was found as the most common and frequent nuisance for dog owners and non-dog owners (Fielding 2008a). In our study sites, nuisances related to free-roaming dogs, such as feces on the street and spilling of garbage, were more often mentioned, and barking was mainly a nuisance for non-dog owners and North American tourists. We found inconsistency in that although most dog owners (82%) let their dogs roam free, only 17% of villagers openly agreed with allowing village dogs to roam free. Villagers possibly answered in terms of what was considered to be appropriate to the outside world, rather than in terms of what they believed, which can occur with in-person surveys (Leggett 2003).

Perceptions of the Dog-Keeping System by Villagers and Tourists

Despite differences in dog-keeping practices, the perceptions of the villagers did not differ among villages. Different to Fielding, Samuels and Mather (2002), we did not find any gender difference in opinions about dog reproduction. Villagers were comfortable with the idea of sterilizing female dogs, but less comfortable with the idea of sterilizing male dogs, which agrees with Fielding, Samuels and Mather (2002). Half of the villagers, nevertheless, believed that female dogs should breed at least once in their lifetime. Breeding females, therefore, could be a pre-requisite for sterilization, which also agrees with Fielding, Samuels and Mather (2002), although wanting a dog to breed is different from wanting a dog to "come on heat" (Fielding, Samuels and Mather 2002). Consistent with the explanation given by various villagers, that female dogs deserve to experience mothering, it appears that villagers highly value motherhood, breeding, or both, and that villagers apply human concerns on reproduction to their dogs, which was also reported by Fielding, Samuels and Mather (2002).

Although many tourists suggested sterilization as a solution to dog-related problems, very few dogs were sterilized, probably because the cost of surgery limits its use in coastal villages of Oaxaca. Sterilizations were offered at no cost, however, during the annual dog sterilization campaign by foreign veterinarians, so one would have expected more dogs to have been sterilized, given that most villagers agreed on sterilization. It is possible, therefore, that just as with allowing dogs to roam free, villagers answered in terms of what was considered to be appropriate to outsiders, rather than in terms of what they believed (Leggett 2003).

Dog Welfare

We have three explanations for differences between tourist and farming villages in regard to perceiving dog-welfare problems. First, people in Río Seco suffer a lack of jobs and health services. According to the hierarchy of needs (Maslow 1943), fulfillment of lower-order needs is necessary before higher-order needs are fulfilled. It is possible, therefore, that people in Río Seco have not yet considered dog welfare to be relevant, because their own basic needs are not fulfilled. Second, tourist development and the influence of foreigners may have unbalanced the dog-keeping system in the tourist villages (Figure 2). The availability of food from the tourist industry may be seasonal, and dogs might find it difficult to obtain enough food when tourists are gone. Availability of food, together with a lack of control of the dog population, may result in a large population of poorly fed village dogs that are prone to disease. We did not, however, measure body condition score of the village dogs. Third, it is possible that tourists have influenced villagers' perceptions on the welfare of dogs and the keeping of dogs.

That more North American (67%) and European (58%) tourists perceived problems of dog welfare than Mexican tourists (33%) may be due to a different frame of reference (see Boogaard, Oosting and Bock 2006) based on different economic and socio-cultural backgrounds. Dog-keeping practices in the tourist villages of Mazunte and Puerto Angel most likely failed to meet expectations of foreign visitors, just as American tourists visiting the Bahamas probably got the impression that "Bahamians do not care as much for their pets as they do" (Fielding 2008b, p. 358).

In our study, compared with Plumridge and Fielding (2003), however, more tourists admitted giving food to dogs during their stay (40% compared with 1%), probably because of different tourist types: cruise ship passengers vs. alternative and backpacker tourists, and because tourists in our study had more opportunities to interact with village dogs. Village dogs with poor welfare may contribute to an unpleasant experience, apart from other inconveniences that tourists may face during their stay in a rural coastal area. Tourists' opinions about dogs, therefore, may affect the local economy (Plumridge and Fielding 2003). We did not ask tourists, as Plumridge and Fielding (2003) did, if they owned a dog at home or if they were members of an animal welfare group, which could have also influenced tourists' opinions: pet owners and members of an animal welfare group could be more critical of dog-keeping practices. Boogaard, Oosting and Bock (2006) found that pet owners perceived the quality of life of farm animals less positively than non-pet owners.

Dog Overpopulation and Poisoning

It is evident that dog overpopulation is a problem in the studied villages, as shown by the human:dog ratio and as perceived by villagers and tourists. There is no indication of a cultural opposition to euthanasia, as reported by Hsu, Severinghaus and Serpell (2003) in Taiwan—most villagers agreed on euthanasia for sick dogs. Lack of veterinary services, together with lack of money, however, may account for why dog poisoning was a main cause of deaths in dogs, as seen in the village survey. Furthermore, 17% of villagers agreed on dog poisoning as a control method, whereas only 2.5% (*n* = 6) of respondents in a study in Dominica mentioned poisoning, among other solutions, to deal with animal overpopulation (Alie et al. 2007). It has long been known (WHO 1988) that culling dogs, be it humane or inhumane, is not a long-term solution to control dog populations; where dogs are removed, others migrate into the area to fill the ecological niche (WHO 1988). Rural villages in the coastal region, however, have no strategy or planning to solve their dog-related problems. Poisoning, therefore, is used as a fast, cheap culling method when overpopulation becomes too problematic.

Recommendations

It could become important to improve dog welfare, especially for residents of the tourist villages Mazunte and Puerto Angel. Villagers could benefit tourists and non-dog owners by implementing simple strategies to reduce problems caused by dogs, such as keeping their dogs restrained at night. This is contrary, however, to many villagers' idea of a guard dog. Thus, restraining dogs at night would only work if security in the area also improved.

Efforts to control the dog population in the rural coastal region are aimed at prevention of rabies and protection of wildlife, whereas this study revealed that these problems were mentioned far less by local people than other dog-related problems. The extent of the damage caused by dogs to sea turtles and their eggs is unknown in this area and is a subject for further research. In other coastal areas, such as in the Yucatán Coast of Mexico (personal communication, Eduardo Cuevas, Pronatura) and in Costa Rica (Leslie et al. 1996), up to 30% of nests are predated by dogs.

A next step in the search for solutions to dog-related problems would be to involve villagers. There is an opportunity to involve villagers in cooperating with governmental entities or NGOs, if these organizations also target the dog-related problems that villagers and tourists experience, and if opinions of villagers are taken into account when choosing methods to control the dog population.

Acknowledgements

Fieldwork for this study was made possible thanks to the Wageningen University Scholarship Program for Master Studies. We wish to thank all the staff at Centro Mexicano de la Tortuga for their logistical support, and the respondents of the villager and tourist surveys for their willingness to participate in this study. The first author thanks David Oseguera Montiel for his valuable help during fieldwork. We thank Antonio Ortega Pacheco, Akke van der Zijpp, Anthony Podberscek, and two anonymous referees for their thoughtful comments on previous drafts of this article. We thank Michael Grossman for editing the article, and Katarina Belovradová for helping us to produce Figure 1.

References

Acosta-Jamett, G., Cleaveland, S., Cunningham, A. A. and Bronsvoort, B. M. D. 2010. Demography of domestic dogs in rural and urban areas of the Coquimbo region of Chile and implications for disease transmission. *Preventive Veterinary Medicine* 94(3-4): 272–281.

Alie, K. A., Davis, W., Fielding, W. J. and Galindo-Maldonado, F. 2007. Attitudes towards dogs and other "pets" in Roseau, Dominica. *Anthrozoös* 20: 143–154.

Boitani, L., Ciucci, P. and Ortolani, A. 2007. Behaviour and social ecology of free-ranging dogs. In *The Behavioural Biology of Dogs*, 147–165, ed. P. Jensen. Wallingford, UK: CABI.

Boletín Estadistico (report). 2006. Indicadores básicos de la actividad turística delestado de Oaxaca. Secretaría de Turismo. Oaxaca, México.

Boogaard, B. K., Oosting, S. J. and Bock, B. B. 2006. Elements of societal perception of farm animal welfare: A quantitative study in The Netherlands. *Livestock Science* 104: 13–22.

Borgal, A. B. 2001. League assists MVMA with spay and neuter program for strays in Mexico. *Our Four-Footed Friends* 98:1.

Burns, G. L. 2003. When wildlife tourism goes wrong: A case study of stakeholder and management issues regarding dingoes on Fraser Island, Australia. *Tourism Management* 24: 699–712.

Butler, J. R. A. and Bingham, J. 2000. Demography and dog–human relationships of the dog population in Zimbabwean communal lands. *The Veterinary Record* 147: 442–446.

CONANP. 2007. Inter-American Convention for the Protection and Conservation of Sea Turtles Mexico (report). 2007. Secretary of Natural Resources and the Environment, National Fisheries and Aquaculture Commission of Mexico (SEMARNAT).

Coppinger, R. and Coppinger, L. 2001. *Dogs: A Startling New Understanding of Canine Origin, Behavior, and Evolution.* New York: Scribner.

Eilers, C. H. A. M., Koops, W. J., Udo, H. M. J., van Keulen, H. and Noordhuizen, J. P. T. M. 2001. Iguana production in Central America: Prospects and constraints based on stakeholders' perceptions. *Outlook on Agriculture* 30: 187–194.

Fielding, W. J. 2008a. Dogs: A continuing and common neighborhood nuisance of New Providence, The Bahamas. *Society & Animals* 16: 61–73.

Fielding, W. J. 2008b. Attitudes and actions of pet caregivers in New Providence, The Bahamas, in the context of those of their American counterparts. *Anthrozoös* 21: 351–361.

Fielding, W. J., Samuels, D. and Mather, J. 2002. Attitudes and actions of West Indian dog owners towards neutering their animals: A gender issue? *Anthrozoös* 15: 207–226.

Foucat, V. S. A. 2002. Community-based ecotourism management moving towards sustainability, in Ventanilla, Oaxaca, Mexico. *Ocean & Coastal Management* 45: 511–529.

Fraser, D. 2008. Toward a global perspective on farm animal welfare. *Applied Animal Behaviour Science* 113: 330–339.

Grennan, E. H. and Fielding, W. J. 2008. Tourists' reactions to non-human animals: Implications for tourist–animal research in the Caribbean (report). Pegassus Foundation.

Hsu, Y., Severinghaus, L. L. and Serpell, J. A. 2003. Dog keeping in Taiwan: Its contribution to the problem of free-roaming dogs. *Journal of Applied Animal Welfare Science* 6: 1–23.

INEGI. 2005. Conteo de población y vivienda 2005. Instituto Nacional de Estadística e Informática de México.

IUCN. 2010. IUCN Red List of Threatened Species. Version 2010.4. <www.iucnredlist.org>. Accessed January 11, 2011.

Kitala, P., McDermott, J., Kyule, M., Gathuma, J., Perry, B. and Wandeler, A. 2001. Dog ecology and demography information to support the planning of rabies control in Machakos District, Kenya. *Acta Tropica* 78: 217–230.

Leggett, C. G. 2003. Social desirability bias in contingent valuation surveys administered through in-person interviews. *Land Economics* 79: 561–575.

Leslie, A. J., Penick, D. N., Spotila, J. R. and Paladino, F. V. 1996. Leatherback Turtle, Dermochelys coriacea, nesting and nest success at Tortuguero, Costa Rica, in 1990–1999. *International Journal of Turtle and Tortoise Research* 2 :159–168.

Macpherson, C. N. L., Meslin, F. X. and Wandeler, A. I. 2000. Dog ecology and population biology. In *Dogs, Zoonosis and Public Health*, 17–50, ed. N. L. Calum. New York: CABI.

Maslow, A. H. 1943. A theory of human motivation. *Psychological Review* 50: 370–396.

Orihuela, T. A., and Solano, V. J. 1995. Demographics of the owned dog population in Miacatlan, Mor. Mexico. *Anthrozoös* 8: 171–174.

Ortega-Pacheco, A., Rodriguez-Buenfil, J. C., Bolio-Gonzalez, M. E., Sauri-Arceo, C. H., Jimenez-Coello, M. and Forsberg, C. L. 2007. A survey of dog populations in urban and rural areas of Yucatan, Mexico. *Anthrozoös* 20: 261–274.

Ortolani, A., Vernooij, H. and Coppinger, R. 2009. Ethiopian village dogs: Behavioural responses to a stranger's approach. *Applied Animal Behaviour Science* 119: 210–218.

Plumridge, S. and Fielding, W. J. 2003. Reactions of American tourists to roaming dogs in New Providence, Bahamas. *Anthrozoös* 16: 360–366.

Poss, J. E. and Bader, J. O. 2007. Attitudes toward companion animals among Hispanic residents of a Texas border community. *Journal of Applied Animal Welfare Science* 10: 243–253.

R Development Core Team. 2010. R: A language and environment for statistical computing. R Foundation for Statistical Computing, Vienna, Austria.

SEMARNAT and CONANP. 2006. Convención Interamericana para la Protección y Conservación de las Tortugas Marinas México, Segundo Informe Anual in Secretaría de Medio Ambiente y Recursos Naturales y Comisión Nacional de Pesca y Acuacultura.

Siegel, S. and Castellan, N. J. 1998. *Non-Parametric Statistics for the Behavioral Sciences.* New York: McGraw Hill.

Slater, M. R. 2001. The role of veterinary epidemiology in the study of free-roaming dogs and cats. *Preventive Veterinary Medicine* 48: 273–286.

SSA. 2001. Programa de acción: Rabia. Secretaría de Salud, Mexico.

Udo, H. and Cornelissen, T. 1998. Livestock in resource-poor farming systems. *Outlook on Agriculture* 27: 219–224.

Valadez-Azúa, R. and Mestre-Arrioja, G. 1999. Años de oscuridad. In *Historia del Xoloitzcuintle en México*, 99–111. México, DF: Museo Dolores Olmedo-UNAM.

WHO. 1988. Report of WHO consultation on dog ecology studies related to rabies control in WHO/Rab.Res./88.25, World Health Organization.

Learn. Lead. Achieve.

Humane Society University

is exclusively dedicated to human-animal studies. Learn to be a better advocate and further your career by enrolling in one of our programs.

Masters Degrees • Graduate Certificates
Bachelor of Science Degrees
Continuing Education • Professional Development

For more information, visit **humanesocietyuniversity.org** or contact **info@humanesocietyuniversity.org.**

Humane Society University
2100 L Street, NW
Washington, DC 20037
p 202.676.2390
f 202.778.6147

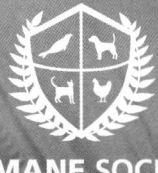

HUMANE SOCIETY
UNIVERSITY™

ANTHROZOÖS   VOLUME 25, ISSUE 1   REPRINTS AVAILABLE   PHOTOCOPYING   © ISAZ 2012
PP. 93–109   DIRECTLY FROM   PERMITTED   PRINTED IN THE UK
THE PUBLISHERS   BY LICENSE ONLY

The Coldest Dog and Pony Show on Earth: Animal Welfare on the First Expeditions to Reach the South Pole

Sarah L. Wilks

Social and Sustainability Research Group, School of Law, University of Western Sydney, New South Wales, Australia

Address for correspondence:
Dr. Sarah Wilks,
School of Law,
University of Western Sydney,
Locked Bag 1797,
Penrith, NSW 2751,
Australia.
E-mail: s.wilks@uws.edu.au

ABSTRACT The expeditions to reach the South Pole mounted by Scott, Amundsen, and others between 1901 and 1912 have attracted considerable scholarly effort. These expeditions all took draught animals, which were key to the success or failure of the missions. Much of the literature in this field is highly partisan, focusing on the relative merits of Scott and Amundsen: the fates of their animals have received little attention except as ammunition for one side or another of this very polarized discourse. This paper describes the treatment of the dogs and ponies taken as draught animals on the expeditions led by Scott and Amundsen. These expeditions were planned such that animals would be used to pull sledges and slaughtered when required for food, or when the food for the animals ran out. Each of these expeditions is shown to have engaged in cruel practices and to have caused some animals extreme suffering. Scott's and Amundsen's management of their animals are compared. Amundsen kept close oversight of the care of the animals whereas Scott tended to delegate, with the results that on occasions Scott's animals did not receive timely attention and suffered as a result. Scott had reservations about using dogs because he viewed them mainly as intelligent companion animals. He had difficulties viewing dogs as working animals that might suffer, or as potential food, but no apparent reservations about using ponies in such ways. Amundsen's attitudes towards the dogs on his expedition and the animals' welfare outcomes are closely examined in this paper in the light of previous contentions that Amundsen was a serial animal abuser. While Amundsen also saw dogs as companions, he viewed them as draught animals and/or food sources as he felt his circumstances warranted. It is shown that outrage at the fates of Amundsen's dogs rests within past hagiographic endeavors in addition to modern western beliefs that dogs are pets, not draught animals; and from Western attitudes towards the consumption of dog flesh.

Anthrozoös DOI: 10.2752/175303712X13240472427519

Keywords: Amundsen, Antarctica, eating dog meat, Scott, working dogs

 The expeditions to the South Pole mounted by Scott, Shackleton, Amundsen, and others between 1901 and 1912 captured, and retained, the public imagination. Since Cook's first crossing of the Antarctic Circle and his subsequent circumnavigation of Antarctica between 1772 and 1775, many explorers had dreamed of reaching the South Pole. None succeeded until Amundsen's successful journey in 1911. The South Pole was also reached a few weeks later by Scott's party, all of whom perished during the return journey to their base. Their deaths so captured the public imagination that, when the news of the polar party's deaths reached the outside world, "We landed to find the Empire—almost the civilised world—in mourning ... " (Cherry-Garrard 1922).

This so-called "Heroic Age" of South Polar exploration (1901–1912) has stimulated a great deal of scholarly and populist effort. The activities of the explorers were captured by photography and/or expedition artists, and many of the expeditioners kept journals and diaries. A large quantity of other source materials exists, which has been extensively studied. In addition, many of the explorers published accounts of their travels upon their return (Scott's account was published posthumously, in 1913). From these and other sources, researchers have sought to explain, comment upon, make sense of, balance the respective worth of and on occasion adulate or denigrate the explorers. In particular, Scott's heroism during his South Polar journey was taken as a given for some fifty years afterwards. A wave of iconoclasm that dates from quite early and reasoned questioning (Hayes 1928), but which peaked in a full-frontal offensive (Huntford 1979), has since questioned the heroic myth. By the 1980s, Scott was portrayed by some as indecisive, bumbling, and incompetent, and Amundsen elevated to hero status in the process. Recently, other workers (e.g., Solomon 2001; Fiennes 2003; Jones 2003; Murray 2008) have sought to re-balance this view: Fiennes' 2003 book is dedicated to "the families of the defamed dead." These opposing findings by workers with different paradigms and agendas, but the same, finite pool of primary sources, will no doubt see-saw for years to come. It is not the intention of this paper to generate ammunition for either side of this contested subject but to offer a balanced view of the ways the explorers treated their animals. In this author's opinion, both Scott and Amundsen were unusual and imperfect men who accomplished astounding things and each bore the impression of his era, social background, and country.

Scott, Shackleton, and Amundsen all took draught animals with them. Surprisingly little scholarship has examined the fates of these animals, although the explorers wrote many words in their journals about the animals that traveled alongside them. They all intended to "use up" the lives of some (or all) of their animals, by using them to haul sledges prior to slaughtering them either for food or when the animals' food ran out.

On most occasions that the presence of animals has been referred to by researchers, their presence is part of an argument developed to demonstrate one explorer's superiority. For example, a repeated theme in the (anti-Scott) literature has been whether Scott actually believed that man-hauling was so noble he was willing to forego draught animals (although, curiously, authors in this camp never question why then did Scott bring any dogs at all?); or whether his experience on his first Antarctic expedition had "turned him off" dog-driving; or whether Scott was simply not adequately prepared for the journey because he was not knowledgeable about dog-handling. Some authors have reported details of parasitology (Campbell 1981) or pathogens (Falckh 1987) from a veterinary viewpoint, but besides Mason's 1979 account of the ponies taken on the *Nimrod* and *Terra Nova* expeditions, which was aimed at younger readers, few authors have commented on the welfare of the animals themselves. An exception is Murray's 2008 publication entitled "The use and abuse of dogs on Scott's and Amundsen's South Pole expeditions."

In this paper, the fates of the animals involved in some of the early Antarctic expeditions are described from an animal welfare perspective. Animals suffered greatly on all of the expeditions, which were characterized by varying degrees of animal welfare concern, efforts, and competency. Finally, a commentary upon Murray's 2008 contention that Amundsen was a serial animal abuser will be offered, with the conclusion that, besides beating Scott to the South Pole, Amundsen's offense was actually to use dogs in what to modern Western perceptions are non-traditional ways (i.e. for motive power and food).

The present analysis draws mainly upon the accounts written by Amundsen and Scott, focusing upon the *Terra Nova* and *Fram* (1910–1912) expeditions. Both men kept diaries and these, along with accounts written by other travelers, have been studied.

At this point in their lives, both Scott and Amundsen had considerable experience of long polar journeys and therefore were well acquainted with the conditions that the members of their teams, human and non-human, would face. As expedition leaders, Scott and Amundsen bore responsibility for planning and execution, including for the well-being of the animals in their charge. Both Scott and Amundsen had previously visited Antarctica, and both had dog-driving experience. Solomon's (2001) finding that the weather conditions on the barrier in Antarctica are far more extreme than conditions in the Arctic is relevant here, as Scott's previous dog-driving experiences were in Antarctica while Amundsen, although having greatly more experience with dogs than Scott, had gained his experience in the climatically more moderate Arctic.

During their expedition planning processes, both Amundsen and Scott consulted accounts of previous expeditions, that is, Scott's 1901–1904 *Discovery* and Shackleton's 1907–1909 *Nimrod* voyages *inter alia*, and Amundsen in particular seems to have consulted Shackleton's *Nimrod* account with a view to informing his own project. Scott's experiences of dog handling on *Discovery* also clearly affected his planning for his second expedition, as will be discussed in greater detail later in this paper. A brief overview of the *Discovery* and *Nimrod* expeditions is given below for the purpose of providing context.

Background: The Expeditions and Their Animal Members
Discovery 1901–1904

On Scott's 1901–1904 *Discovery* expedition, he took 45 "terrified" sheep and 23 dogs as deck cargo. The dogs had been transported from Russia and were loaded with the sheep onto *Discovery* in New Zealand. The dogs were chained up amidships, on chains sufficiently short to prevent the dogs from having physical contact with their neighbors. The sheep were penned on coal sacks on deck, out of reach of the dogs. No shelter from the elements was provided for the animals. En route from New Zealand to Antarctica, Scott worried that the *Discovery* might encounter heavy weather, in which case: " ... all our sheep and possibly many of the dogs would have been drowned" (Scott 1905, p. 87). The sheep were slaughtered at sea about three weeks after leaving New Zealand. All the dogs arrived alive in Antarctica.

The dogs were put to work hauling sledges only after considerable difficulties, caused mainly by a lack of experience or understanding of dogs. On November 2, 1902, Scott, Shackleton, and Wilson harnessed all the dogs for a long journey to break a trail towards the South Pole. The dogs were to be fed dried fish, which had a low fat content and was therefore not suited to their needs. Once underway, the dogs' performance began to fade. By November 17, Wilson wrote in his diary that the dogs were tiring and the men had begun hauling the sledges as well. By November 24, the dogs were " ... very weary indeed ... the driving of them has become a perfectly beastly business ... " (Wilson 1966, p. 217): they were "dead beat" on November 25. On November 27, he wrote: "We came on a mile this morning but the dogs required too much beating and eventually gave up trying to pull." On November 30, Wilson wrote: "The amount of shouting and beating that the dogs want before they will do any work at all is soul sickening."

The dogs were forced to continue through beatings to " ... get them on, yard, by yard" and when one dog collapsed again, he was described as " ... preferring to be dragged to keeping on his feet" (Wilson 1966, p. 220). When four of the dogs began passing blood, the food was suspected to be tainted. One dog died and was found post mortem to have had acute peritonitis. The surviving dogs apparently picked up a little after eating the carcass. In early December, a decision was made to "feed up 8 or 9 of the best dogs on the others" and by mid December the "best" dogs were improving while the rest: " ... are getting daily thinner and weaker ... " (p. 225). One by one the remaining animals sickened and died or were killed. On December 29 one dropped dead in harness, and on the 31st another died from "sheer weakness."

The expedition turned back on December 31, 1902. The next day, Wilson wrote that the " ... dogs are terribly weak and of very little use. Another dog dropped on the march today, too weak even to walk" (Wilson 1966, p. 232). This animal was left to be attacked and eaten by the other dogs. On January 2, 1903, another dog died and a further two animals were close to death. On the 3rd, "Two more dropped in their traces ... " another one on the 6th, yet another on the 11th and by the 14th it was finally recognized that the remaining two "utterly useless" dogs were so debilitated that they were not ever going to recover, let alone work, and (Doctor) Wilson killed them by using a sharp scalpel to stab through their hearts.

Scott, Wilson, and Shackleton were very deeply affected by the suffering they had caused the *Discovery* dogs. Wilson was haunted by it and Shackleton would later unsuccessfully rely on ponies rather than dogs on his *Nimrod* expedition, with the probable loss of being the first to reach the South Pole (Amundsen 2010, p. 214). Scott's reaction to this is discussed in further detail below.

Nimrod 1907–1909

Shackleton's experiences with Scott on *Discovery* clearly informed his own effort to reach the South Pole. He wrote: " ... my hopes were based mainly on the ponies. Dogs had not proved satisfactory ... " (Shackleton 1909, p. 21), and that he brought dogs " ... as a standby in the event of the ponies breaking down" (p. 165). Shackleton took 15 Manchurian ponies on the 1907–1909 *Nimrod* expedition towards the South Pole, which eventually stopped 180 kilometers short. During the 70-day voyage to Antarctica the ponies were not able to lie down. The vessel was overloaded and only had three feet of freeboard, with the result that the ponies were constantly exposed to the water and weather. Only eight ponies survived this voyage and were unloaded onto Antarctica "in bad condition" (p. 87): one animal had been essentially flayed by constant knocking and rubbing against the sides of the stalls while at sea and was shot upon landing. Within six weeks of their arrival in Antarctica, four more ponies had died of preventable causes, having eaten substances that they should have been prevented access to. Shackleton also took nine dogs, of which eight survived the trip south, unsheltered on deck. Upon landing, the dogs were tied up to rocks and left for two days in bad weather with no shelter or food, causing the death of another dog.

On October 29, 1908, Shackleton set out towards the South Pole with all four ponies, planning to eat their flesh at some point on the expedition: " ... when the ponies go under" (Shackleton 1909, p. 276). One rapidly became lame: within ten days, two ponies were not feeding well and all were "losing condition" (p. 271). On November 21, the first pony was shot: he had been "struggling painfully along," followed a week later by the next, an animal which had been suffering with snow-blindness (p. 294). By November 30, one of the remaining ponies was " ... very shaky and seemingly on his last legs" and both were snow-blind (p. 296). The weak pony was "quite finished" the next day and was shot. The remaining pony " ... was lonely. He whinnied all night for his lost companion ... " (p. 299) and survived another five days' hauling prior to falling into a deep crevasse on December 7. The men then continued south-wards, pulling the sledge themselves.

Terra Nova and Fram 1910–1912

By 1909 there were rumors of several impending expeditions aiming to be the first to reach the South Pole. Scott's *Terra Nova* expedition set out first. Like *Discovery*, this expedition had a scientific program in addition to forming an attempt to "conquer" the South Pole.

Amundsen's original plans were known only to a very few people. Leaving Norway in 1910 with the stated aim of reaching the North Pole (reportedly reached by Peary and/or Cook in 1909), Amundsen sailed to Madeira whereupon he announced, to the surprise of his crew and financiers, that he would actually attempt to beat Scott's party to the South Pole. It was, ret-rospectively, obvious from his preparations that Amundsen had intended to journey south all along. Amundsen later admitted to his patron (the distinguished Norwegian polar expert Fridtjof Nansen) that he had been planning to go to the South Pole since September 1909 (Langner 2007, p. 114).

Scott was only informed that there was a rival expedition at a late stage and decided that he would not deviate from his original plans, essentially declining to race. Amundsen's "de-ception" was not easily forgiven, at least in the eyes of the British—"Naturally the sympathies of Englishmen at least will be with Captain Scott ... " (The Times 1911)—or by some of Amund-sen's more influential compatriots (Bomann-Larsen 1995).

Scott's decision to rely mainly upon ponies rather than dogs for his push towards the South Pole during *Terra Nova* was probably made for the reasons given in his published ac-count of the earlier *Discovery* expedition, and based upon the suffering of the dogs he had wit-nessed on that expedition. In an oft (partially) quoted passage, Scott notes that there are two ways to use dogs on expeditions of this nature: " ... they may be taken with the idea of bring-ing them all back safe and sound, or they may be treated as pawns in the game, from which the best value is to be got regardless of their lives" (Scott 1905, p. 340). If it were intended to save the lives of the dogs, Scott believed that " ... properly organised parties of men will per-form as extended journeys as teams of dogs ... " (p. 341). If it were intended to use the dogs by feeding them to other dogs, then Scott acknowledged that the radius of action would be increased, but expressed his reluctance for work of this nature: "One cannot calmly contem-plate the murder of animals which possess such intelligence and individuality ... " before finally concluding that, if the end was found to justify the means, the important thing was to avoid unnecessary pain: " ... to suddenly and painlessly end the life of an animal which has been well fed and well cared for is not cruelty." Later in the passage, under the running heading of "our sad experience," Scott notes his relief on commencing man-hauling the next season (the dogs having all died in the first season), knowing that the horrors of the previous season would not recur. Scott's subsequent paragraph has been on occasion quoted, minus context, to serve arguments that Scott had over-heroic aspirations about the nobility of man-hauling versus using draught animals: it is the paragraph where Scott in effect says that working without dogs, and man-hauling the sledges instead, is a more honorable way to proceed and gain a more satisfying achievement. However, it is clear, in the context of the preceding paragraphs, that Scott said this because he found the suffering of the dogs distressing. Scott saw dogs as individual animals with intrinsic worth and generally liked dogs as pets, and he personally struggled with the idea of using up dogs' lives in order to further the mission. If they were to be so used, then he stated that cruelty via under-feeding or over-working should be avoided and the dogs should be killed painlessly. Given his experiences with the *Discovery* dogs described above, Scott probably would not have found it easy to envisage cruelty-free outcomes.

How Far Can We Trust *post-facto* Accounts?

The potential for *post-facto* polishing of narratives in order to present a more acceptable face can be clearly seen from the *Discovery* accounts. Wilson's *Discovery* diary was probably not intended for publication: Wilson wrote expressly to his family in his *Terra Nova* diary: " ... this journal ... keep it from any chance of being used for publications ... " (Wilson 1972, p. 191). Scott worked up his published *Discovery* account from his original diaries. While Scott's published version mentions poor welfare outcomes for the dogs, it does not approach the level of detail given by Wilson and discussed above. Were it not for Wilson's account, the full extent of the suffering of the dogs would not be clear.

Shackleton also had opportunity to gloss-over or massage descriptions of the fates of his animals, and indeed may have done so. However, the remaining tales indicate that many of these animals suffered extreme agonies and endured hideous deaths, although Shackleton seems to have taken some thought for animal welfare. Care was taken to administer a clean head shot away from the other animals, in order not to upset the survivors and he wrote that, " ... we had the satisfaction of knowing that the animals had been well fed and well treated up to the last, and that they suffered no pain" (Shackleton 1909, p. 290), although snow blindness in humans is reportedly extremely painful.

During the *Terra Nova* and *Fram* expeditions, both Scott and Amundsen kept diaries with a view to lucrative publication deals upon their return. During the last few days prior to his death, Scott seemed to be very confident that his diaries would be found, writing his famous "*Message to the British Public*" and many letters to friends and supporters. Based upon the recovered diaries, the posthumous "*Scott's Last Expedition*" (Scott 1913) was a lightly edited version of Scott's actual words.

Amundsen's account, "*The South Pole,*" was based upon his diaries and was published in the English language in 1912, after translation of the hurriedly written Norwegian original. Unlike Scott's generally inviting prose in his diaries, Amundsen's original diaries (Amundsen 2010) are relatively terse and less accessible. It is likely that Amundsen viewed his diaries as very private and not to be published (Kløver 2010), not least because he provided a great deal of detail about an embarrassing and painful personal problem.

The circumstances of authorship of the published *Fram* and *Terra Nova* accounts, namely that Amundsen could have edited in order to justify his actions or manipulate his account in order to present his desired version of events, while Scott obviously could not, do not necessarily invalidate the analytical approach used in this paper. However, this potential limitation does need to be examined. Amundsen may have colored his account in his 1912 book where Scott could not, but to what extent does this affect a reasonable, non-partisan reading of the two sources? The answer to this may depend on the material under consideration. While the contention that Amundsen may have retrospectively portrayed himself in a flattering light has an irresistible pull, this effect cannot do much to soften some of the very stark differences between the ways Scott and Amundsen treated their animals. An example of this can be seen in the (independently verifiable) accounts of the ways the two teams' animals were transported to Antarctica.

Scott took 19 Manchurian ponies and 33 Siberian dogs on the *Terra Nova* expedition. The dogs and ponies had been selected for him by an agent who knew very little about horses. The agent relied upon the advice of the horse trader, who had clearly enjoyed the better end of the bargain, and the ponies were neither young nor in good health. During the 100 days the ponies were at sea, they were forced to stand. Scott wrote: "It seems a terrible ordeal for these poor beasts to stand this day after day for weeks together, and indeed though they continue to feed well the strain quickly drags down their weight and condition; but nevertheless the trial cannot be gauged from human standards ... " (Scott 2006, p. 13). Seventeen ponies survived this journey to reach Antarctica.

Scott described his arrangements for the transport of the dogs thus:

> Upon the coal sacks, upon and between the motor sledges and upon the ice-house are grouped the dogs, thirty-three in all. They must perforce be chained up ... their position is not enviable. The seas continually break on the weather bulwarks and scatter clouds of heavy spray ... The dogs sit with their tails to this invading water, their coats wet and dripping. It is a pathetic attitude, deeply significant of cold and misery; occasionally some poor beast emits a long pathetic whine. The group forms a picture of wretched dejection; such a life is truly hard for these poor creatures. (Scott 2006, p. 14)

Amundsen did not take any ponies on his expedition, relying solely on dogs for motive power. Ninety-seven "Eskimo" dogs were sourced from Greenland. The dogs were housed for the journey south on a loose deck built over the existing deck, the intervening air space providing insulation from extremes of temperature. This was taken up and cleaned regularly. Awnings and wooden paneling provided shade and shelter. The dogs were divided into squads of about ten and each assigned to a keeper "with full responsibility for their animals and their treatment." The dogs were washed and brushed regularly and: "We get fonder and fonder of them every day and the love is mutual. They shriek for joy when they see us ... " (Amundsen 2010, p. 48). After a period of habituation, the dogs were allowed run of the ship except when being fed. Two dogs were lost overboard and female puppies were disposed of during the voyage. Amundsen's diary makes frequent reference to the well-being of the dogs, including, for example, Amundsen's decision to try feeding the dogs a higher fat diet when the dried fish-based diet appeared not to be enough: "It is amazing to see how the dogs have improved ... as I thought, they lacked fat ... " (p. 67).

There is thus no reasonable doubt that Amundsen's dogs were better cared for, at least during transportation to Antarctica than Scott's animals, no matter who was alive or dead and able or not to edit their diaries prior to publication.

Scott's *Terra Nova* Animals at Work

The transport of Scott's ponies and dogs to Antarctica has been described above. Once ashore, the animals were given a period of habituation prior to commencing operations. During early depot-laying expeditions, it was noticed that the ponies did not cope well with blizzard conditions, one becoming a "miserable scarecrow" (Scott 2006, p. 119). Less than a week later, one pony fell down and was immediately set upon by a dog team, and two sticks were broken on the dogs' backs while trying to separate the dogs from the pony (p. 123).

Out on the trail in January 1911, a dog began coughing and died within minutes of an unknown cause. Although Scott mentions, periodically (Scott 2006, e.g., pp. 107, 133), that he thought the dogs were being underfed, he makes no record of any corrective actions. Recounting an incident in which a previously friendly dog had bitten him, Scott mused upon dog nature, appearing to reconsider his stance against the consumptive use of dogs:

> Hunger and fear are the only realities in dog life: an empty stomach makes a fierce dog. There is something almost alarming in the sudden fierce display of natural instinct in a tame creature. Instinct becomes a blind, unreasoning, relentless passion ... It is such stern facts that resign one to the sacrifice of animal life in the effort to advance such human projects as this. (Scott 2006, p. 116)

By late February, the dogs were "thin as rakes," and two ponies had died due to exposure and hard work. On February 28, 1911, after an enforced stop due to a blizzard, when the blankets were taken off the ponies it was seen that they were "terribly emaciated." The pony which had been attacked earlier by the dog team was in a "pitiable" condition and died later that night (Scott 2006, p. 138). Days later, a party with four ponies was caught on breaking ice: one pony was lost and three were left on a floe overnight. The next day, while Scott's men were attempting to rescue them, two animals ended up in the water, which was full of hunting killer whales (p. 141). One pony was inefficiently bludgeoned to death with an ice pick because it was being/would have been eaten alive by the killer whales. Oates, the expedition's horse handler, remarked at the time, "If I have to kill another animal like that I will be sick ... " and declined to kill the second pony, handing the ice pick over to another man prior to advising him where to strike the pony.

Meanwhile at the expedition headquarters, another dog had died of unknown causes, and a pony had gradually sickened until he was too weak to stand, eventually being "put out of his misery." Facing the polar winter and the (southern) spring trip to the Pole, there were ten ponies left. Two more dogs died of unknown causes over the winter.

After starting for the Pole in the next (Antarctic) spring, the ponies began to fade sooner than had been anticipated (Scott 2006, p. 323) and on November 24, 1911, the first pony was shot: he had been fading for the previous four days and Scott wrote that it was "merciful" to have ended his life (p. 329). The pony's carcass was fed to the dogs and four days later another pony was shot, providing more food. On December 1, another pony was shot. Scott noted that all were failing but that they would outlast the amount of fodder the expedition carried. Another pony was shot on December 2, and another on the 3rd. By this time all the men were " ... consuming horse flesh and thoroughly enjoying it" (p. 338). The remaining ponies were shot on December 9, having finished the last of the fodder. Although Scott wrote that, "... the ponies were quite done, one and all, they came on painfully slowly a few hundred yards at a time ... " he also said that it was "hard to have to kill them so early" (p. 342): he does not specify if this is concern for the expedition, regret at having under-catered for the ponies, or because he liked the animals. In the event, the exhausted ponies hauled sledges on their last march with no food (one man, Wilson, gave his biscuit ration to his hungry pony and marched without food himself). It is surprising, given Scott's distressing *Discovery* experiences of working his dogs to death, and his personal observations of the effects of inadequate diet and extreme weather upon the animals, that he was not more alert to distress among the ponies during the *Terra Nova* operations.

Unlike Scott's deliberations on the morality of using dogs, there was apparently no questioning of the "using up" of ponies' lives in this way. The ponies were to pull sledges until the terrain, or the end of their rations, prevented them from being of any further use, at which point they were to be slaughtered. This seems to be a reflection of Scott's beliefs about what dogs and horses were "for": horse-drawn transport was still the norm in England at the time of the *Terra Nova* expedition. In contrast, there was (and had been for decades) widespread feeling within Britain that using dogs as draught animals was inherently cruel, and it is probable that Scott was influenced by this. In Europe, there were surviving practices of using dogs as draught animals: besides the tradition of using dogs to pull sledges in snowy regions, dogs were used to pull milk carts and the like in the Netherlands and Switzerland, and would be used to pull machine gun carts in Belgium and ammunition carts in Italy during the Great War (Burns 2008). However, in Britain the use of dogs as draught animals had been proscribed by law in 1854, ostensibly on nuisance grounds but certainly owing much to animal welfare activism (Pemberton and Worboys 2007). This legislation was re-enacted in 1911 in the *Protection of Animals Act* on explicit animal welfare grounds (Radford 2001).

Amundsen's *Fram* Animals at Work

After an abortive first start (it turned out to be too early in the season and the weather was inclement), Amundsen started towards the pole with five men, and four sledges with 13 dogs apiece. Three dogs were released on the first day because they were not physically up to the job: two eventually found their way home. Four marches later, the party reached a depot and the dogs were given as much seal meat as they were capable of eating. During the two rest days at the depot, "The dogs gnawed and gnawed, storing up strength with every hour that went by" (Amundsen 2008, II, p. 18). Amundsen planned to travel in daily 17-mile marches, less than half the distance he felt they could have done, noting (although surely he had the presence of the rival Scott expedition always in his mind) that it " ... was more important to arrive than to show great speed ... we were interested in seeing how the dogs would manage the loaded sledges. We expected them to do well, but not so well as they did" (p. 20). At the 82°S depot, two dogs were slaughtered and placed into store for the return journey, and again the party took a rest day and the dogs were given all they could eat. By 83°S, another dog had been slaughtered and three had "deserted." Passing 84°S, the party left provisions for five men and 12 dogs, the anticipated size of the return party. At 85°S, and facing a climb up to the polar plateau, 42 dogs remained. On the plateau, 24 dogs were slaughtered. Three sledges pulled by 18 dogs proceeded towards the pole.

The party reached the pole on December 14, 1911. Both dogs and men were suffering from the effects of the cold and altitude. Leaving the pole four days later, 16 dogs remained, three of which were soon fed to the others. By December 28, Amundsen wrote that the dogs were: " ... bursting with health ... howling for joy ... putting on flesh day by day and getting quite fat" (Amundsen 2008, II: p. 143). The polar party returned to base on January 25, 1912, with 11 dogs. Within days the entire party, including 39 dogs, were loaded onboard ship for transport to Hobart, where 21 dogs were given to Mawson for his upcoming Australasian expedition to Antarctica.

Upon Amundsen's announcement that he would try to beat Scott and be the first man to reach the South Pole, and perhaps partially due to perceived deceit on Amundsen's part, a certain amount of media attention and other commentary was focused upon his use of dogs. This was said to be cruel, unnatural and, in the event that Amundsen reached the pole first, would represent a hollow victory. Amundsen was very aware of the existence of perceptions that using dogs on such expeditions was cruel. Upon arrival in Antarctica, Amundsen wrote in his diary:

> ... our transport of these dogs over a distance of 16,000 km in all kinds of weather and practically all temperatures is not just a complete success, but also evidence of special and thoughtful care. A reminder to the many who thought that the expedition would involve animal cruelty from the first to the last. (Amundsen 2010, p. 81)

After his successful return from the pole, Amundsen went so far as to crow in his published account: "I still cannot help smiling when I think of the compassionate voices that were raised here and there—and even made their way into print—about the "cruelty to animals" on board the *Fram*. Presumably these cries came from tender-hearted individuals who themselves kept watch-dogs tied up" (Amundsen 2008, I: p. 60).

Amundsen's Dogs: Ammunition for Revisionist Historians?

Murray (2008) argued that Amundsen was guilty of a degree of ruthlessness and brutality towards his dogs that Scott would not have stooped to, hinting that Amundsen was a serial animal abuser who retrospectively endeavored to portray himself as an animal lover. Bolstering his argument with quotations from Amundsen's 1912 book *"The South Pole,"* Murray states that Amundsen subjected his dogs to extreme suffering throughout the expedition, listing examples in support of this thesis, including that unwanted puppies were disposed of and that many adult dogs were killed or died of exhaustion throughout the expedition. In addition, Murray claims that, far from being the animal lover he (Amundsen) professed himself to be, Amundsen was uncaring about the state of his dogs, rather too willing to eat them, and bloodthirsty in his approach to the native wildlife. These accusations will be further explored below.

With respect to the disposal of unwanted pups, Amundsen is certainly not alone. During the *Discovery* expedition, Scott wrote: "Nell has added seven to the puppy population ... We shall probably reduce this to four or five ... " Female dogs come into estrus twice a year. Litter sizes vary but six is a reasonable starting point for rough calculations, and both Scott and Amundsen mentioned litters of this size. Each breeding female could potentially contribute 12 dogs per year. The additional food and care demands resulting from unrestrained increase in the dog population would have proven problematic to both leaders. The only practical way to control the size of the dog packs was either to limit the female population by killing some pups, or not to have brought females at all, in which case there would be no means to increase the size of the dog pack if needed.

Quoting Amundsen[1], Murray says:

> Adult dogs were killed or died of exhaustion throughout the expedition. On a depot-laying journey, one called Thor was killed with an axe. Another, Lurven, "reduced to skin and bones ... fell down on the march and died on the spot ... he pulled and pulled until he died." (Amundsen's words in double quotation marks, Amundsen 1976, I: p. 242)

There is no doubt that some of the dogs taken on Amundsen's second depot-laying excursion in 1911 (the sledging season prior to his attempt to reach the pole) suffered terribly. Buoyed by a far easier and smoother first depot-laying trip than he had anticipated: " ... my admiration for these splendid animals rose to a pitch of enthusiasm ... I think the dogs showed on this occasion that they were well suited to sledging on the Barrier ... brilliant result ... " (Amundsen 2008, I: pp. 220–221), Amundsen planned a second trip. However, even before they had gone as far as the first depot, some dogs were showing signs of exhaustion due to cold weather and overloading: " ... the dogs were beginning to be stiff and sore-footed and it was hard work to get them started in the morning" (p. 231). An unexpected cold snap affected men and dogs alike, and at 81°S, after a rest, Amundsen went on with five "very thin, and apparently worn out" (p. 234) dogs, having sent one back due to a large raw patch from his harness. Amundsen had hoped to get to 83°S but: "Our dogs, especially mine, looked miserable—terribly emaciated. It was clear they could only reach 82°S at the farthest. Even then the homeward journey would be a near thing" (p. 236). The dogs on Amundsen's team foundered: relating this as " ... the only dark memory of my stay in the south ... " Amundsen unsuccessfully tried to whip the dogs into motion then, leaving his sledge at the depot, assigned them to other teams for the trip home. Subsequent cold weather compounded the animals' exhaustion until one dog, Thor, was unable to rise one morning and, in the absence of firearms, was dispatched with an axe. Thor was later found to have had a large quantity of pus in his chest. Later that day, one of Amundsen's original dog team dropped dead in harness, followed by another dog the next day. The remaining two dogs " ... had to be put an end to that day; it was a shame to keep them alive any longer" (p. 244). In his sledging diary for this period, Amundsen wrote: " ... this tour has unfortunately cost the lives of eight of our best dogs ... probably due to the unusual cold ... we worked all the time in severe cold ... average temperature has been about –40°C ... " (Amundsen 2010, p. 146).

This excursion echoes Scott's 1902 *Discovery* experiences: both were disastrous for the dogs concerned because neither leader had anticipated the very extreme cold on the barrier. Amundsen later wrote: "Tempted by the favorable outcome of our former trip, we put too much on our sledges this time—on some of them, in any case. Mine was overloaded. I had to suffer for it afterwards—or rather, my noble animals did" (Amundsen 2008, I: p. 227). With respect to Thor, Amundsen wrote remorsefully: "I feel it yet when I think of Thor ... uttering his plaintive howls on the march. I did not understand what it meant ... " (p. 238). To Murray, Amundsen's statement that " ... in normal circumstances I loved my dogs ... The daily hard work and the object I would not give up had made me brutal, for brutal I was when I forced those five skeletons to haul that excessive load" (p. 238) is unsatisfactory, and Murray invokes other possible explanations including Amundsen's views of masculinity and of modern, technological outlooks. Citing a biographer who hinted that in his later years, Amundsen simply lost the plot as he struggled to keep his place in a world that wanted younger heroes, Murray speculates that Amundsen later suffered psychoses in part due to this brutalization of animals. However, although by 1927 (i.e., 15 years after the *Fram* expedition) Amundsen's behavior had become increasingly erratic and had been the subject of "hush-up" attempts by senior statesmen (Bomann-Larsen 1995), there is no indication that Amundsen was suffering incipient psychoses while he was in Antarctica.

Amundsen, in fact, did not drive a dog team in Antarctica ever again. He distributed his remaining dogs amongst other drivers. He does not explain this decision other than as a cryptic aside in his sledge diary to the effect that he did not "dare" drive dogs again (Amundsen 2010, p. 197), and that he would act as the lead runner ahead of the caravan in the spring journey towards the pole.

During his disquisition, Murray commits several instances of that which he accuses those denigrating Scott to be guilty of: selective quotations, or quotation of material that in the original documents is clearly embedded in a context which does not support the conclusions Murray attempts to draw from it. For example, Murray says:

> Early in his book Amundsen made it clear that he compelled absolute submission: "the dog must understand that he has to obey in everything" (Amundsen 1976, I: p. 58). Later the author explained that he was aided by the fact that his "Eskimo" dogs had a deeper fear of him than domestic dogs, the result of their stronger "instinct of self-preservation" and their dependence on him for food. (pp. 196–197, Amundsen's words in double quotation marks)

Read uncritically, these quotations impute a character to Amundsen that is not evident when the context of the quote is examined. At the first page reference cited by Murray above, Amundsen is expressing his astonishment at Scott's and Shackleton's dismissal of dogs as useful in Antarctic journeys and making the point that dog-driving requires understanding of the dogs' nature:

> There must be some misunderstanding or other at the bottom of the Englishmen's estimate ... Can it be that the dog has not understood his master? Or is it the master who has not understood his dog? The right footing must be established from the outset; the dog must understand that he has to obey in everything, and the master must know how to make himself respected ... (Amundsen 2008, I: p. 58)

In addition, immediately prior to the second page reference given by Murray, Amundsen had written at some length upon the character and behavior of his so-called Eskimo dogs (Amundsen 2008, I: p. 195), going on to opine that the Eskimo dog is more closely related to the wolf than are domestic dogs. Amundsen's view was that the Eskimo dog was less domesticated: "We must not call the Eskimo dog slow to learn because he cannot sit up and take sugar when he is told: these are things so widely separated from the serious business of his life that he will never be able to understand them, or only with the greatest difficulty." Amundsen then stated his belief that Eskimo dogs had a greater instinct for self-preservation and a more pronounced "pack" mentality than domestic dogs:

> Among themselves the right of the stronger is the only law. The strongest rules, and does as he pleases undisputedly: everything belongs to him. The weaker ones get the crumbs.
>
> ... The weaker, with his instinct of self-preservation, seeks the protection of the stronger. The stronger accepts the position of protector, and thereby secures a trusty helper, always with the thought of one stronger than himself.
>
> ... The dog has learnt to value man as his benefactor, from whom he receives everything necessary for his support. (p. 196)

What Amundsen is saying here is that his relationship with the dogs was on terms that the dogs, with their hard-wired inclinations to a pack hierarchy, could understand. Amundsen was literally, in the eyes of the pack, the top dog, or in his own words, the "protector." Thus, when he goes on to say:

> As a consequence of this, his respect for his master is far greater than in our domestic dog, with whom respect only exists as a consequence of the fear of a

> beating. I could without hesitation take the food out of the mouth of any one of my twelve dogs; not one of them would attempt to bite me. And why? Because their respect, as a consequence of the fear of getting nothing next time, was predominant. (Amundsen 2008, I: p. 197)

he is demonstrating his understanding of what makes the Eskimo dogs "tick" (while perhaps demonstrating an incomplete understanding of more domesticated dogs). This passage alone indicates that Murray's depiction of Amundsen as a person who had no empathy with the dogs is not defensible.

Later in the article, Murray refers to dogs being repeatedly flogged and physically punished, although this imputes a tenor to Amundsen's book that does not exist. Indeed, reference to the original text quoted by Murray to make this "point" (Amundsen 1976, II: p. 16) shows that on the occasion cited, Amundsen was trying to restore order after one dog (Hai) snatched another dog's (Rap) rations. Amundsen intervened immediately:

> Meanwhile, I had witnessed the whole scene, and before Hai knew anything about it, I was upon him in turn. I hit him over the nose with the whip-handle and tried to take the pemmican from him, but it was not so easy. Neither of us would give in, and soon we were both rolling over and over in the snow struggling for the mastery. I came off victorious after a pretty hot fight, and Rap got his dinner again. (Amundsen 2008, II: p. 16)

Amundsen's decision to roll around fighting in the snow to retrieve a piece of food from the sharp teeth of a semi-wild dog rather than just giving Rap another portion (the party was well-supplied at that point) illustrates two things: the pack mentality of the dogs (do anything you can get away with to a weaker individual while respecting those who are stronger) and Amundsen's understanding that he had to intervene because had the thief got away with it, then that dog would have challenged other dogs and Amundsen in the future.

It is instructive to compare this instance of Amundsen physically punishing a dog with an incident related by Scott during the *Discovery* expedition. One day, the dog pack turned upon a particular individual and "murdered" the dog. While Scott was waiting for a break in the weather to get " ... these bloodthirsty wretches chained up ... " there was another attack and " ... another poor beast lay mangled on the ice-foot." Scott described his course of action the next day: " ... one by one, they were led out and severely chastised in front of their victims" (Scott 1905, p. 190). It is of course entirely pointless and potentially cruel to attempt to discipline a dog the day after it has committed a transgression and Scott himself was aware that the dogs didn't understand why they were being whipped: " ... the dogs evidently didn't know what it was all about ... " However, Scott continued beating the animals anyway because: " ... the punishment helped to relieve our righteous indignation ... " (Scott 1905, p. 191).

Comparing Scott's and Amundsen's reactions to disorder in the ranks of the dogs, it is not hard to see which of the two men had the greater understanding of the animals, and which of the two was engaging in unthinking cruelty.

Dogs on the Menu

A further point of attack from Murray relates to Amundsen's planned slaughter and consumption of some dogs on the Polar trip. While planning, Amundsen had noted the: " ... obvious advantage that dog can be fed on dog. One can reduce one's pack little by little, slaughtering the feebler ones and feeding the chosen with them" (Amundsen 2008, I: p. 58).

During the polar expedition, Amundsen's party arrived on the plateau four days ahead of schedule and had been looking forward to fresh meat: " … the thought of the fresh dog cutlets that awaited when we got to the top made our mouths water" (Amundsen 2008, II: p. 57). They had already selected individuals for this cull: " … a difficult problem to solve, so efficient were they all." Later the next day, when Amundsen was at his usual evening task of arranging the tent and starting the cooking, he wrote:

> … the part of my work that went more quickly than usual that night was getting the Primus started, and pumping it up to high pressure. I was hoping thereby to produce enough noise to deaden the shots that I knew would soon be heard — twenty four of our brave companions and faithful helpers were marked out for death …

> Each man was to kill his own dogs …

> The pemmican was cooked remarkably quickly that evening, and I believe I was unusually industrious in stirring it … I am not a nervous man but I must admit I gave a start. (pp. 62–63)

The entrails and trimmings went straight to the other dogs, who " … spent the night in eating; we could hear the crunching and grinding of their teeth … " (Amundsen 2008, II, p. 64), but the men's mouths were no longer watering with anticipation: "The holiday humor that ought to have prevailed in the tent that evening did not make its appearance; there was depression and sadness in the air — we had grown so fond of our dogs … we could not fall upon our four-footed friends and devour them before they had had time to grow cold" (p. 64). However, by the next day, as one member of the party butchered the carcasses into more appetizing cuts, Amundsen was clearly feeling more cheerful: "Great masses of beautiful fresh red meat, with quantities of the most tempting fat, lay spread over the snow … the delicate little cutlets had an absolutely hypnotising effect as they were spread out one by one over the snow … " (p. 65): the cutlets were eaten with " … lightning-like rapidity."

To many contemporary Western eyes, eating dog and other "non-food" meats is a taboo only to be broken under circumstances of exceptional hardship (Simoons 1994). Dog and horse meat were eaten throughout the German Empire in the years leading up to the First World War (*The New York Times* 1907). Cat meat was offered for sale by English butchers during the First World War (Arthur 2003, p. 67). Faced with increasing meat shortages during the Second World War, German authorities sanctioned the supply of dog meat and other non-traditional meats including wolves, foxes, bears, and badgers, for human consumption (*Time Magazine* 1940).

However in some cultures, eating dog is not unusual: areas of south-east Asia, Africa, and Polynesia have long traditions of dog consumption. These customs are deeply embedded in the cultural histories of the groups concerned but can be highly contentious when seen through Western eyes. A recent case of a man of Tongan origin, living in New Zealand, who followed the customary Tongan practice of killing and cooking his dog and then serving it to his guests (*CNN World* 2009), sparked widespread condemnation. In Nigeria, dog meat is eaten with relish in several provinces, although this practice is viewed by some non-Nigerian people as disturbing and disgusting (Nairaland 2007). Chinese authorities did their best to suspend the offering of so-called "fragrant meat" (dog) in restaurants during the 2008 Beijing Olympics, in concession to Western concerns about the consumption of dog meat (Dickie 2008). Podberscek's 2009 study of dog and cat consumption in South Korea noted the high level of international opposition to these practices, as well as an apparently staunch defense of this aspect of their cultural identity even by South Korean people who would not themselves consume these animals.

As Serpell (2009) and others have pointed out, people culturally accustomed to treating dogs as family members may find the killing and consumption of dogs repugnant. It is thus tempting to dismiss Murray's outrage that Amundsen planned his expedition in such a way as to "use up" his dogs as a manifestation of contemporary Westernized attitudes towards "food" and "non-food" animals (although analogous outrage on behalf of Scott's ponies is lacking). However, as demonstrated by the discussion above, and reading this in mind of Murray's stated aim (i.e., to "restore some balance to one part of the long record of adulation of Amundsen and denigration of Scott"), it is clear that Murray is prosecuting war on Amundsen in the tradition of past hagiographic efforts. Murray's thesis, at least with respect to Amundsen's "troubled and contradictory attitudes towards his animals," is not defensible. While Amundsen did take a very utilitarian view of the dogs, as essential tools for use in the achievement of his goal, he generally took extremely good care of these tools. Whatever Amundsen's other personal failings, there is no evidence of general callousness and cruelty of the sort inferred by Murray on Amundsen's expedition. Neither is there any evidence that Amundsen as expedition leader and manager tolerated the sort of acts of animal cruelty by omission, carelessness, or ignorance that characterized Scott's expeditions, some of which have been described above. One suspects that besides his original sin of beating Scott to the South Pole, what Amundsen has really done wrong here is to offend modern sensibilities with respect to "food" species: yet as has been noted, what is an acceptable "food" or "non-food" species can vary with culture, time, and place.

Conclusions

Considerable animal suffering was associated with the early expeditions towards the South Pole. Amundsen relied solely upon dogs for motive power and Scott relied upon dogs and ponies. Both Scott and Amundsen wrote extensively about their animals, claimed that they were animal lovers, and expressed regret when their animals suffered. Both explorers planned to slaughter at least some of their draught animals during the expeditions. Amundsen planned to kill some dogs later in his journey and to feed the meat to the remaining dogs. He and his men also ate dog meat. Scott planned to travel as far as he could with the ponies, limited by either the amount of fodder they had or the amount of work the ponies could do before they were worked out, and then to shoot them. He and his men consumed some of the horse meat.

Amundsen saw himself as a dog-lover and viewed his dogs as sometimes companions, sometimes working animals, and sometimes food. He took great care that the dogs had an appropriate diet and adequate shelter, and demonstrated his personal knowledge and understanding of dogs and dog handling on many occasions. In most instances when an animal became sick or was obviously suffering, he ensured that the animal was appropriately treated or euthanized promptly. Amundsen expressed regret for the ending of dogs' lives, and affection and respect for the animals, on many occasions. When caught out by unexpectedly severe weather on one of his early journeys, resulting in extreme suffering and the subsequent deaths of several dogs, Amundsen was sufficiently affected by his actions that he did not trust himself to drive dogs again. He walked/ran much of the way to the South Pole instead, a round journey of approximately 2,800 kilometers.

Scott also saw himself as a dog-lover and struggled with the idea of dogs in roles other than as man's best friend. Due to this, and distressed by his part in causing extreme suffering to several dogs during his first Antarctic expedition, Scott planned to preserve the lives of the dogs on his second expedition by relying on ponies instead, with the dog teams used as accessory means of transport in relatively non-demanding ways. Despite this reluctance to use up dogs' lives, Scott had no evident problems with the idea of using up ponies' lives. In the case of the ponies, extreme suffering was not necessarily met with appropriate remedial actions, not even timely and humane euthanasia. Scott's general approach to animal care and management was to delegate responsibility, but he failed to personally ensure that the required actions were taken. Thus, while Scott noted, for example, that inadequate shelter for the animals was provided during transport, he did not cause this to be rectified and this led to unnecessary animal suffering.

Acknowledgements

The author thanks Professor Trevor Tansley and the two anonymous reviewers for their many insightful comments.

Note

1. When quoting Amundsen, Murray (2008) relied upon the 1976 facsimile of Amundsen's 1913 book. When quoting Amundsen, I have referred to the 2008 edition. Both books contain two volumes, that is, I and II, and the page numbering is similar but not identical. When quoting Scott with respect to the *Discovery* expedition, I am referring to Scott (1905): "The Voyage of the 'Discovery'" Volume I. When quoting Scott on the Terra Nova expedition, I am referring to Scott (2006): "Journals," which contains the text of "*Scott's Last Expedition*" (1913) in addition to the deletions of some material from Scott's original writings made by the editor of "*Scott's Last Expedition*."

References

Amundsen, R. 1976. *The South Pole: An Account of the Norwegian Expedition in the "Fram," 1910–1912.* Translated by A. G. Chater. St. Lucia: University of Queensland Press (facsimile of original work published in 1912).

Amundsen, R. 2008. *The South Pole: An Account of the Norwegian Expedition in the "Fram," 1910–1912.* Translated by A. G. Chater. London: HURST.

Amundsen, R. 2010. *The South Pole Expedition 1910–1912.* Translated by Z. Støp and J. Brannan. Ed. G. O. Kløver. Oslo: The Fram Museum.

Arthur, M. 2003. *Forgotten Voices of the Great War.* Imperial War Museum. London: Ebury.

Bomann-Larsen, T. 1995. *Roald Amundsen.* Translated by I. Christophersen. Stroud: Sutton Publishing.

Burns, P. 2008. *Dog Carts and the Extinction of Memory.* <www.terriermandotcom.blogspot.com> Accessed January 5, 2011.

Campbell, W. C. 1981. Heartworm in Scott's Antarctic expedition. *American Heartworm Society Bulletin* 7: 5–7.

Cherry-Garrard, A. G. B. 1922. *The Worst Journey in the World.* London: Constable.

CNN World. 2009. Man escapes charges for barbecuing pet dog. <www.articles.cnn.com> Accessed September 10, 2010.

Dickie, M. 2008. Beijing wants dogs off menu during Olympics. <www.ft.com> Accessed January 20, 2011.

Falckh, R. C. F. 1987. The death of Petty Officer Evans. *Polar Record* 23: 397–403.

Fiennes, R. 2003. *Captain Scott.* London: Hodder & Stoughton.

Hayes, J. G. 1928. *Antarctica. A Treatise on the Southern Continent.* London: The Richards Press.

Huntford, R. 1979. *Scott and Amundsen. The Race to the South Pole.* London: Pan.

Jones, M. 2003. *The Last Great Quest. Captain Scott's Antarctic Sacrifice.* Oxford: Oxford University Press.

Kløver, G. O. 2010. Introduction. In *The South Pole Expedition 1910–1912.* R. Amundsen. Translated by Z. Støp and J. Brannan. ed. G. O. Kløver. Oslo: The Fram Museum.

Langner, R-K. 2007. *Scott and Amundsen.* Translated by T. Beech. London: Haus Publishing.

Mason, T. 1979. *The South Pole Ponies.* New York: Dodd, Mead & Co.

Murray, C. 2008. The use and abuse of dogs on Scott's and Amundsen's South Pole expeditions. *Polar Record* 44: 303–310.

Nairaland, 2007. How to cook dog meat for soup (strictly Calabar and Ondo). <www.nairaland.com> Accessed on February 4, 2011.

Pemberton, N. and Worboys, M. 2007. *Mad Dogs and Englishmen.* Basingstoke: Palgrave Macmillan.

Podberscek, A. L. 2009. Good to pet and eat: The keeping and consuming of dogs and cats in South Korea. *Journal of Social Issues* 65: 615–632.

Radford, M. 2001. *Animal Welfare Law in Britain.* Oxford: Oxford University Press.

Scott, R. F. 1905. *The Voyage of the "Discovery." Volume 1.* London: MacMillan.

Scott, R. F. 1913. *Scott's Last Expedition. Volume 1.* London: Dodd, Mead.

Scott, R. F. 2006. *Journals. Captains Scott's Last Expedition.* ed. M. Jones. Oxford: Oxford University Press.

Serpell, J. A. 2009. Having our dogs and eating them too: Why animals are a social issue. *Journal of Social Issues* 65: 633–644.

Shackleton, E. 1909. *The Heart of the Antarctic.* London: Heinemann.

Simoons, F. J. 1994. *Eat not this Flesh. Food Avoidances from Pre-history to Present.* Westport: University of Wisconsin Press.

Solomon, S. 2001. *The Coldest March.* Carlton South: Melbourne University Press.

The New York Times. 1907. Germany's dog meat market. The consumption of canines and horses is on the increase. *The New York Times*, June 23. <www.nytimes.com> Accessed February 4, 2010.

The Times. 1911. The race to the South Pole. *The Times*, March 30. <www.timesonline.co.uk> Accessed October 6, 2010.

Time Magazine. 1940. Germany: Dachshunds are tenderer. *Time Magazine,* November 25. <www.time.com> Accessed February 2, 2010.

Wilson, E. A. 1966. *Diary of the Discovery Expedition to the Antarctic Regions 1901–1904*. ed. A. Savours. London: Blandford Press.

Wilson, E. A. 1972. *Diary of the Terra Nova Expedition to the Antarctic 1910–1912*. ed. H. G. R. King. London: Blandford Press.

ISAZ2012

THE ARTS AND SCIENCES OF HUMAN–ANIMAL INTERACTION

JULY 11TH TO 13TH

MURRAY EDWARDS COLLEGE, CAMBRIDGE, UK

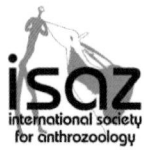

Topics which will be covered include:

* Animals and human-animal interaction in film, television, literature, music and art
* Attitudes to animals and animal issues (contemporary and historical)
* The impact of human-animal interactions on the health and well-being of people and animals
* Cultural studies of human-animal interaction
* Animal welfare and ethical issues

Registration now open. Early bird registration ends March 30th, 2012

2012 marks the 25th anniversary of *Anthrozoös*, Journal of the International Society for Anthrozoology. Join us for this special event in the journal's history.

For further information, go to: www.isaz2012.com

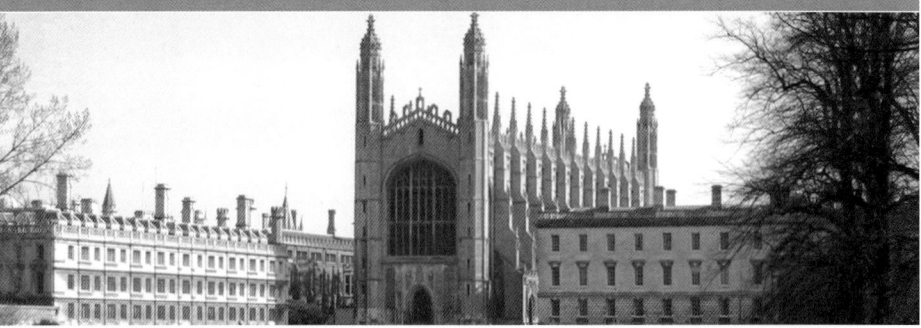

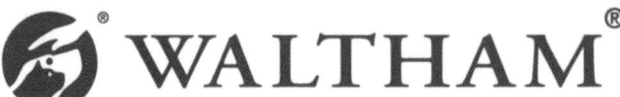

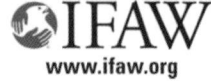

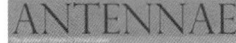

ANTENNAE

ANTHROZOÖS   VOLUME 25, ISSUE 1   REPRINTS AVAILABLE   PHOTOCOPYING   © ISAZ 2012
PP. 111–119   DIRECTLY FROM   PERMITTED   PRINTED IN THE UK
THE PUBLISHERS   BY LICENSE ONLY

Childhood Neglect, Attachment to Companion Animals, and Stuffed Animals as Attachment Objects in Women and Men

M. Rose Barlow, Cory Anne Hutchinson, Kelsy Newton, Tess Grover and Lindsey Ward

Department of Psychology, Boise State University, Idaho, USA

Address for correspondence:
M. Rose Barlow,
Department of Psychology,
Boise State University,
1910 University Dr.,
Boise, ID 83725-1715, USA.
E-mail:
rosebarlow@boisestate.edu

ABSTRACT Childhood neglect has severe, pervasive, negative outcomes that often continue into adulthood. As a potential source of support for both children and adults, companion animals (pets) can both give and receive affection and therefore may be sources of healthy attachment for people who were raised in negative situations. Toy stuffed animals, in contrast, can only receive affection but may still be useful as transitional objects, particularly for people who experienced interpersonal neglect in childhood and who are in the midst of a transition away from the family home and into college. The current study examined the relationships among childhood neglect, companion animal attachment, and attachment to toy stuffed animals. Undergraduate participants ($n = 457$) from a large regional university answered questionnaires online. The first hypothesis, that self-reported childhood neglect would be positively related to attachment to companion animals, was supported for women only. Neglected women were more attached to companion animals than were non-neglected women, with a medium effect size. For men, there was no significant effect. The second hypothesis was that childhood neglect would be positively related to attachment to stuffed animals; this hypothesis was not supported. The third hypothesis, that women would be more attached to both companion animals and stuffed animals than would men, was supported. Attachment to companion animals and attachment to stuffed animals were positively related. Results are discussed within a framework of attachment and transitional objects as potential aids to therapy in people who were neglected in childhood.

Keywords: animal attachment, gender, neglect, pets, stuffed animals

Anthrozoös   DOI: 10.2752/175303712X13240472427159

Neglect is perhaps the most common form of child maltreatment, and yet it is one of the least studied. Adults who were neglected in childhood may have difficulties adjusting to major life transitions, such as moving to a new community and entering college. In this study, we examined whether childhood neglect is related to two possible forms of comfort-seeking: relationships with companion animals (pets) and the use of stuffed animals for emotional comfort. The literature in these three areas has so far not been connected. Therefore we will briefly review literature on human–animal interaction, human relationships to stuffed animals, and childhood neglect.

Human–animal interactions (HAI) have been increasingly studied in the past two decades. For many Americans, owning one or more companion animals is a way of life. According to statistics from the American Veterinary Medical Association in 2007, over 37% of US households own at least one dog, and over 32% own at least one cat. The same study reported that almost half of the dog or cat owners considered their animals to be members of the family (AVMA 2007).

Many people believe that relationships between humans and companion animals are beneficial not only to the animal but also to the owner (e.g., Staats, Sears and Pierfelice 2006; Staats, Wallace and Anderson 2008). For example, HAI may be particularly useful to people who experience stigma, such as those recovering from serious mental illness (Wisdom, Saedi and Green 2009). In a sample that included both college students and clients with diagnosed dissociative disorders, participants who had survived severe childhood abuse had particularly strong attachments to animals, indicating a potential coping mechanism (Barlow et al. in press). Companion animal owners have also been shown to have a better survival rate after acute myocardial infarction than non-owners (Friedmann and Thomas 1995), and HAI may directly and positively influence an owner's physiological state, increasing oxytocin levels and affecting social bonding (Nagasawa, Mogi and Kikusui 2009), or improving cardiovascular responses to stress (Allen, Blascovich and Mendes 2002).

Most studies of HAI focus on the positive effects of emotional relationships with companion animals (e.g., Winefield, Black and Chur-Hansen 2008). These emotional benefits have been conceptualized within an attachment framework. As it was originally developed, attachment theory explains the relationship between infants and caregivers from an evolutionary survival perspective (Shaver and Mikulincer 2009). Some characteristics of attachment have been applied to relationships between companion animals and humans (see Kurdek 2009a for a critical summary of this application).

The term "attachment" is often applied loosely when developing measures of HAI. It is unclear whether traditional attachment theory relates directly to HAI or whether these interactions diverge from the theory in important ways (Crawford, Worsham and Swinehart 2006). Beck and Madresh (2008) studied attachment styles in relationships among humans as well as in human–companion animal relationships. Their participants were more likely to be securely attached to companion animals than to romantic partners, rating relationships with companion animals to be less anxious and to contain less avoidance than interpersonal romantic relationships. The authors suggested that human–animal relationships contained the same basic structure or styles as human–human relationships. However, within each person, attachment styles may be very different when comparing attachment to a single romantic partner (or to multiple other humans) with attachment to nonhuman animals (Beck and Madresh 2008). Sable (1995) reported that companion animals may serve as a replacement for, or an extension of, attachment to humans. This finding is the subject of some disagreement, however, in that Cohen (2002) found that people who were more attached to companion animals were no more likely to lack close human relationships, though HAI may meet relationship intimacy and affection needs.

Companion animals are capable of both giving and receiving affection (Albert and Bulcroft 1988) and therefore HAI may be perceived to be as important as human social support. Kurdek (2009a) found that adults were likely to turn to their animals in a time of emotional need instead of to their parents, friends, or children; the only exception was romantic partners. Particularly in students making a transition to college, this support may be especially important as social groups change and human family members are further away. Staats, Wallace and Anderson (2008) found that avoidance of loneliness was the most salient reason for keeping a companion animal in both college students and in middle-aged community members. They also reported that companion animals can help bridge the gap between family life and social networks in college life by providing support for coping, even in students who still lived with their parents. They concluded that companion animals provide important social support, particularly in people who are unmarried, and pointed out that the role of a companion animal in one's life may change over time, particularly during life transitions.

In addition to differences in person-to-person attachment versus human–animal attachment, differences in degree of companion animal attachment may be linked to individual difference variables such as level of dissociation (Brown and Katcher 2001; Barlow et al. in press). Demographic variables may also predict companion animal attachment. In one study (Bodsworth and Coleman 2001), families with children had the lowest attachment to their animals, while singles or families without children reported more attachment. In contrast, Cohen (2002) found that family constellations and other interpersonal relationships had no effect on attachment to companion animals.

Gender differences in HAI have been found in some cases. Herzog (2007) emphasized that men and women are generally similar on level of attachment to animals, with some studies showing women more attached, but with small effect sizes. Staats, Sears and Pierfelice (2006) found that, while men and women were both likely to have and to value companion animals, they kept animals for different reasons. In their sample of high-functioning and healthy university faculty, women were more likely than men to report social support reasons for having a companion animal, such as reducing loneliness and having someone to help them through hard times. Faculty who were alone or isolated were also more likely to endorse these social support aspects. Men were more likely to report keeping a companion animal for pragmatic reasons, such as exercising with a dog. Both genders reported spending a large amount of time with their companion animals (Staats, Sears and Pierfelice 2006).

While attachment to companion animals has been found to be in many ways similar to attachment to humans, toy stuffed animals have been conceptualized to serve more as a comfort object than as a replacement for human attachment. Feelings towards stuffed animals have not been much studied in adults, especially not in normative populations. Jaffe and Franch (1986) found that 12 of 27 adolescents who were in a psychiatric hospital used stuffed animals to fulfill various important meanings and roles, such as the toy representing an imaginary friend or the person who gave them the toy, the toy acting as a soothing tool, or the toy simply serving as a decoration. In one case study, a woman was found with 17 stuffed animals near and on her bed (Stern and Glick 1993). She reported that the stuffed animals were her friends. In another case study, a 50-year-old man used a hand-held puppet to talk to his doctor, in order to psychologically distance himself from his anxiety (Stern and Glick 1993).

Like companion animals (Parish-Plass 2008), stuffed animals can also be useful in therapy with children who have been abused or neglected and who therefore have impaired abilities in forming secure attachment relationships. Neglect is an unfortunately common occurrence that can be studied in college populations. One study found rates of physical neglect to be nearly 18%, in a sample of over 1000 residents of a US metropolitan area (Scher et al. 2004). Depending on how neglect is conceptualized and measured, it may range as high as 30% (Straus and Savage 2005). No studies that we know of have examined both neglect and stuffed or live animal attachment, though animal abuse has been shown to be an indicator of child maltreatment (e.g., Ascione et al. 2003; DeGue and DiLillo 2009).

The current study examined the relationships between stuffed animal attachment, companion animal attachment, and self-reported childhood neglect. Parish-Plass (2008) proposed that forming secure attachment relationships with companion animals may help children learn how to have healthier relationships in adulthood. More research is needed in this area, particularly given Beck and Madresh's (2008) proposal that attachment to people and attachment to animals may draw on different working models. During the transition out of a family home and into a college dormitory, stuffed animals such as teddy bears may provide an important source of unconditional and controllable comfort.

Because of these overall benefits of companion animals and stuffed animals, it is reasonable to infer that similar benefits would be gained by individuals who may have been neglected and who are now forming new relationships, specifically college students. This population is undergoing a transition to a new lifestyle which, in most cases, coincides with living outside the family home for the first time and changing social support networks (Staats, Wallace and Anderson 2008). It may also involve living away from the family and its animals.

The relationships between neglect and companion animal attachment, and between neglect and stuffed animal attachment, have been little studied to date. The purpose of this study was to examine these relationships. The first hypothesis was that experiencing childhood neglect would be associated with higher attachment to companion animals. The second hypothesis was that neglect would be positively related to stuffed animal attachment, based on previous literature about the need for a transitional object. The third hypothesis was that women would be more attached to companion animals and to stuffed animals than would men (see Herzog 2007).

Methods
Participants
The study involved 457 students at a large regional university in Idaho, USA, aged from 18 to 62 years, sampled from lower-division undergraduate psychology courses. They consisted of 248 females and 194 males. (Fifteen participants did not report their gender and were not included in the gender analyses.) The mean age was 22.7 years ($SD = 6.79$) and there was no age difference between males and females. Most participants were in their first year of college. Eighty-two percent described themselves as White or European American, 4% as Asian or Asian American, 1% as American Indian/Alaska Native, 1% as Black or African American, less than 1% as Native Hawaiian/Pacific Islander, and 6% as biracial or multiracial. The remaining participants did not answer this question. This distribution is characteristic of the location in which data were collected—according to 2010 US Census data, the state of Idaho is 89.1% White, 1.2% Asian, 1.4% American Indian or Alaska Native, 0.6% Black, 0.1% Native Hawaiian or other Pacific Islander, and 2.5% biracial or multiracial (United States Census Bureau 2010).

Measures

The Pet Attachment and Life Impact Scale (PALS), developed by Cromer and Freyd (2004), was used to measure pet attachment. It is a 39-item, self-report scale that covers various aspects of relationships with companion animals, including relational aspects (e.g., "A pet completes the family"); emotional benefits (e.g., "Pets provide stability for me"); and negative impacts ("Having a pet is a financial hardship") (reverse scored). Answers are given on 5-point Likert-type scales (1 = Not at all or Never; 5 = Very much or Always), with higher scores representing more attachment to companion animals. It was developed through empirical studies, originally based on a factor analysis of responses from 350 undergraduate students and later refined and validated on a sample of 651 undergraduate students from a different university on the East Coast. The Cronbach's alpha for the PALS in this East Coast sample was 0.97 (Cromer and Barlow, unpublished data), which compares favorably with the Cronbach's alpha of 0.89 for the Lexington Attachment to Pets Scale (Johnson, Garrity and Stallones 1992). In the current study of 457 students, the Cronbach's alpha for the PALS was 0.95. The PALS correlates well with several existing measures of HAI (rs from 0.61 to 0.81; Cromer and Barlow, unpublished data).

Attachment to stuffed animals was measured with the Stuffed Animal Attachment Questionnaire (SAQ; Cromer and Freyd 2004), a 20-item, self-report questionnaire using 4-point Likert-type scales for responses: from 0 (Not at all true) to 3 (Very true). It inquires into participants' attitudes towards stuffed animals as heirlooms and keepsakes, as having a personality, and as capable of providing love. Examples of items are: "My stuffed animals have personalities all their own," "Stuffed animals can give you love," and "I somehow feel safer with a stuffed animal." In this study, the Cronbach's alpha for the SAQ was 0.77.

Additionally, we measured neglect with the Multidimensional Neglectful Behavior Scale, developed by Straus, Kinard and Williams (1995). This 20-item self-report questionnaire quantifies neglect of children's basic needs by primary caregivers. It has four subscales and these encompass neglect of emotional needs ("My parents did not tell me they loved me"), cognitive needs ("My parents did not read books to me"), supervision needs ("My parents did not care if I got in trouble at school"), and physical needs ("My parents did not give me enough to eat"). Each item is assessed on a 4-point scale: from 1 (strongly disagree) to 4 (strongly agree). The scale has both good internal reliability and construct validity (Straus, Kinard and Williams 1995).

Procedure

Participants filled out self-report measures online in exchange for partial credit towards a course requirement. All participants gave informed consent, and the study was approved by the school's Institutional Review Board. Participants could refrain from answering any question without penalty, and completion of the questionnaire was not timed. After completion, participants were debriefed as to the nature of the study.

Results

Companion animal attachment and stuffed animal attachment were positively correlated ($r = 0.24$, $p < 0.001$). This was also the case when looking at each gender separately: women ($r = 0.20$, $p < 0.01$); men ($r = 0.21$, $p < 0.01$). People who had at least one stuffed animal were more attached to companion animals ($n = 292$, mean PALS = 88.13, $SD = 26.9$) than were people who did not own any stuffed animals ($n = 98$, $M = 71.99$, $SD = 29.97$) ($F_{(1, 388)} = 24.93$, $p < 0.001$, $d = 0.57$ [medium effect size]).

Scores on the Multidimensional Neglectful Behavior Scale can range from 20 (never any neglect; strongly disagree with all neglect items) to 80 (strongly agree with all neglect items). Scores in our sample ranged from 20 to 74. Neglect scores had a unimodal distribution with a positive skew, with relatively few high values. There was no significant difference between males and females in regard to amount of reported parental neglect in childhood, either on the total neglect scale or on any of the subscales ($ps > 0.05$). For subsequent analyses, participants were divided into two groups: those that had experienced any neglect, and those who had not. Scores of 40 and below were characterized as "no neglect" and those above 40 were coded as "neglected." This division resulted in approximately 82% of participants being placed in the "no neglect" group. The "no neglect" group had 153 males and 201 females. The "neglected" group had 30 males and 34 females.

A 2 (gender: male, female) $\times$ 2 (neglect: any, none) factorial MANOVA was conducted, with the PALS and SAQ scores as dependent variables. Covariance of observations was not equal across groups; however, there was a large n with relatively equal groups of males and females. As MANOVA is robust against violations of assumptions, analysis proceeded.

The first hypothesis was that self-reported childhood neglect would be related to higher PALS scores. This was not supported (Wilks' $\lambda = 0.99$, $F_{(2, 340)} = 1.17$, $p > 0.05$, observed power = 0.255). However, looking at women only, neglected females were more attached to companion animals ($n = 34$, mean PALS = 99.27, $SD = 26.77$) than were females who did not experience neglect ($n = 175$, $M = 88.26$, $SD = 25.80$, $t_{(204)} = -2.10$, $p < 0.05$, $d = 0.42$ [medium effect size]).

The second hypothesis was that self-reported childhood neglect would be related to higher SAQ scores. This was not supported (Wilks' $\lambda = 0.99$, $F_{(2, 340)} = 1.17$, $p > 0.05$, observed power = 0.255).

The third hypothesis was that women would have higher scores than men on both the PALS and SAQ. This was supported (Wilks' $\lambda = 0.93$, $F_{(2, 340)} = 13.52$, $p < 0.001$, Partial eta-squared = 0.074, observed power = 0.998). Follow-up univariate ANOVAs revealed that gender was related to PALS score ($F_{(1, 341)} = 23.02$, $p < 0.001$): women were more attached to companion animals ($M = 89.93$, $SD = 25.99$) than were men ($M = 75.32$, $SD = 29.08$, $d = 0.53$). Gender was also related to SAQ score ($F_{(1, 341)} = 8.96$, $p < 0.01$): women were more attached to stuffed animals ($M = 40.21$, $SD = 7.84$) than were men ($M = 38.24$, $SD = 4.95$, $d = 0.41$). Women also reported having more stuffed animals than did men, with a mean of 3.5 ($SD = 1.84$) stuffed animals owned by women versus a mean of 1.00 ($SD = 1.46$) stuffed animals owned by men ($d = 1.51$).

Discussion

Our first hypothesis, that neglect would be positively correlated with companion animal attachment, was partially supported. We predicted this result based on prior literature that shows that animals can be an important source of social support during stressful times, particularly for people who do not have that support from other humans. Neglected women showed moderately more attachment to companion animals than did non-neglected women, with a medium effect size. No significant effect was found in men, though their numbers were slightly smaller. Note that the number of women reporting neglect in this sample was also relatively small ($n = 34$), suggesting that this effect merits further exploration and replication in larger samples.

The second hypothesis, that self-reported childhood neglect would be related to higher attachment to stuffed animals, was not supported. However, it seems that people who have stuffed animals may be more attached to companion animals than are those with no stuffed animals. The current study builds on past work by Cromer and Freyd (2004). A question naturally arising from this line of research is, if people are attached to both, does it represent a generalized love of animals, desire for tactile contact, or different types of emotional relationships? Future research should address these questions.

If tactile comfort is a key component, perhaps benefits can be found with simple stuffed animal interventions. A recent intervention called "Huggy Puppy" suggests that traumatized children in particular may benefit from toy stuffed animals (Sadeh, Hen-Gal and Tikotzky 2008). Children between two and seven years old who had been displaced to a camp during a war showed faster reduction of stress responses when they were given a stuffed animal and encouraged to care for it, compared with children who did not receive a stuffed animal (Sadeh, Hen-Gal and Tikotzky 2008). This work, along with the current study, implies that stuffed animals may in some cases be a viable replacement for, or addition to, HAI, and may provide some of the same benefits.

The third hypothesis was that women would be more attached to companion animals and to stuffed animals than would men. This hypothesis was supported, with small to medium effect sizes. This finding is consistent with what Herzog found in his 2007 review: when studies do find a gender difference in attachment to companion animals, it is small and in the direction of women being more attached than men. It is possible that these results are reflective of larger gender roles in which men are not demonstrative of affection, and in fact our study did find that women had more stuffed animals than did men (with a very large effect size). In an earlier study, Cromer and Freyd (2004) found that women had many more stuffed animals than did men, with a mean of nearly 17 stuffed animals owned by women and a mean of fewer than four for men. However, these researchers did not report any gender analysis of attachment levels.

Research comparing HAI with human–human relationships needs to take more notice of important variables in the inter-human relationships. For example, in several studies, Zeifman and Hazan (2008) found that attachment relationships between adult romantic partners can take up to two years to develop all the functions of attachment (proximity-seeking, separation distress, secure base, and safe haven). Conversely, in examining attachment dimensions of avoidance and anxiety, Beck and Madresh (2008) suggested that the type of animal can play a role in distinguishing different types of human–animal attachment; for example, dog owners and cat owners reported different attachment styles with their pets. Further research should also more carefully delineate different elements of attachment, as Kurdek (2009b) has found that safe haven, one defining element of attachment, may be only a minor component of human attachment to companion animals in college students.

Stuffed animals are common transitional objects for children and adolescents, but it is important to remember that they may not always serve as attachment objects (Cromer and Freyd 2004). Stern and Glick (1993) argued that more adolescents are attached to stuffed animals than not. This comfort could otherwise be derived from companion animals, but college dormitories and rental housing often exclude animals of any sort. These findings point the way for applied studies in which stuffed animals are studied as aids in psychotherapy, self-regulation, and coping.

Recent work (Barlow et al. in press) suggests that attachment to companion animals and to stuffed animals may follow a similar pattern and be associated with similar traits, such as dissociation. In that study, attachment to companion animals was positively correlated with attachment to stuffed animals, in samples including college students and patients diagnosed with mental illness. This is consistent with the findings of Cromer and Freyd (2004) and with those of the current study, in which companion animal attachment and stuffed animal attachment were positively and significantly related. It appears that both toy and live animals may serve a similar purpose in some situations.

The current finding that neglected women reported more attachment to companion animals than did non-neglected women deserves further examination and replication. There may be certain aspects of neglect or trauma for which stuffed animals or other transitional objects are a useful component of therapy, even in adulthood, but little research has been done in this area. One limitation of the current study is that neglect is difficult to study, especially with retrospective self-report questionnaires. Future research extending the current results should examine different ways of conceptualizing or measuring neglect. In addition, the current sample had low rates of reported neglect, especially among men. These limitations of sample size preclude the use of some statistical techniques and limit the generalizability of the findings.

More extensive research is also needed in order to address the limitations of our sample in terms of age and ethnic diversity, and more applied studies could also examine interactions with animals (live or toy) in real-time. HAI and stuffed animal attachment may represent important covariates with social support. Applications of this research could help survivors of abuse and neglect make life transitions more smoothly.

Acknowledgement
The authors thank Joanna Lahey for helpful feedback on earlier drafts of this article.

References

Albert, A. and Bulcroft, K. 1988. Pets, families, and the life course. *Journal of Marriage and the Family* 50: 543–552.

Allen, K., Blascovich, J. and Mendes, W. B. 2002. Cardiovascular reactivity in the presence of pets, friends, and spouses: The truth about cats and dogs. *Psychosomatic Medicine* 64: 727–739.

American Veterinary Medical Association. 2007. *US Pet Ownership and Demographics Sourcebook.* Schaumburg, IL: Author.

Ascione, F. R., Friedrich, W. N., Heath, J. and Hayashi, K. 2003. Cruelty to animals in normative, sexually abused, and outpatient psychiatric samples of 6- to 12-year-old children: Relations to maltreatment and exposure to domestic violence. *Anthrozoös* 16: 194–212.

Barlow, M. R., Cromer, L.D., Caron, H. P. and Freyd, J. J. in press. Comparison of normative and diagnosed dissociation on attachment to companion animals and stuffed animals. *Psychological Trauma: Theory, Research, Practice, and Policy.*

Beck, L. and Madresh, E. A. 2008. Romantic partners and four-legged friends: An extension of attachment theory to relationships with pets. *Anthrozoös* 21: 43–56.

Bodsworth, W. and Coleman, G. J. 2001. Child–companion animal attachment bonds in single and two-parent families. *Anthrozoös* 14: 216–223.

Brown, S. and Katcher, A. 2001. Pet attachment and dissociation. *Society & Animals* 9: 25–41.

Cohen, S. P. 2002. Can pets function as family members? *Western Journal of Nursing Research* 24: 621–638.

Crawford, E. K., Worsham, N. L. and Swinehart, E. R. 2006. Benefits derived from companion animals, and the use of the term "attachment." *Anthrozoös* 19: 98–112.

Cromer, L. D. and Freyd, J. J. 2004. Stuffed animals, pets, and dissociation. Poster presented at the American Association for the Advancement of Science annual conference, February 12 to 16, 2004, Seattle, USA.

DeGue, S. and DiLillo, D. 2009. Is animal cruelty a "red flag" for family violence? Investigating co-occurring violence toward children, partners, and pets. *Journal of Interpersonal Violence* 24: 1036–1056.

Friedmann, E. and Thomas, S. A. 1995. Pet ownership, social support, and one-year survival after acute myocardial infarction in the Cardiac Arrhythmia Suppression Trial (CAST). *The American Journal of Cardiology* 76: 1213–1217.

Herzog, H. 2007. Gender differences in human–animal interactions: A review. *Anthrozoös* 20: 7–21.

Jaffe, S. and Franch, K. 1986. The use of stuffed animals by hospitalized adolescents: An area for psychodynamic exploration. *Journal of the American Academy of Child Psychiatry* 25: 569–573.

Johnson, T. P., Garrity, T. F. and Stallones, L. 1992. Psychometric evaluation of the Lexington Attachment to Pets Scale (LAPS). *Anthrozoos* 5: 160–175.

Kurdek, L. 2009a. Pet dogs as attachment figures for adult owners. *Journal of Family Psychology* 23: 439–446.

Kurdek, L. 2009b. Young adults' attachment to pet dogs: Findings from open-ended methods. *Anthrozoös* 22: 359–369.

Nagasawa, M., Mogi, K. and Kikusui, T. 2009. Attachment between humans and dogs. *Japanese Psychological Research* 51: 209–221.

Parish-Plass, N. 2008. Animal-assisted therapy with children suffering from insecureattachment due to abuse and neglect: A method to lower the risk of intergenerational transmission of abuse? *Clinical Child Psychology and Psychiatry* 13: 7–30.

Sable, P. 1995. Pets, attachment, and well-being across the life cycle. *Social Work* 40: 334–341.

Sadeh, A., Hen-Gal, S. and Tikotzky, L. 2008. Young children's reactions to war-related stress: A survey and assessment of an innovative intervention. *Pediatrics* 121: 46–53.

Scher, C. D., Forde, D. R., McQuaid, J. R. and Stein, M. B. 2004. Prevalence and demographic correlates of childhood maltreatment in an adult community sample. *Child Abuse & Neglect* 28: 167–180.

Shaver, P. R. and Mikulincer, M. 2009. An overview of adult attachment theory. In *Attachment Theory and Research in Clinical Work with Adults,* 17–45, ed. J. H. Obegi and E. Berant. New York: Guilford Press.

Staats, S., Sears, K. and Pierfelice, L. 2006. Teachers' pets and why they have them: An investigation of the human–animal bond. *Journal of Applied Social Psychology* 36: 1881–1891.

Staats, S., Wallace, H. and Anderson, T. 2008. Reasons for companion animal guardianship (pet ownership) from two populations. *Society & Animals* 16: 279–291.

Stern, T. and Glick, R. 1993. Significance of stuffed animals at the bedside and what they can reveal about patients. *Psychosomatics: Journal of Consultation Liaison Psychiatry* 34: 519–521.

Straus, M. A., Kinard, E. M. and Williams, L. M. 1995. The Multidimensional Neglectful Behavior Scale, Form A: Adolescent and Adult-Recall Version. Durham: University of New Hampshire. Available from <http://pubpages.unh.edu/~mas2/Mul.htm>.

Straus, M. A. and Savage, S. A. 2005. Neglectful behavior by parents in the life history of university students in 17 countries and its relation to violence against dating partners. *Child Maltreatment* 10: 124–135.

United States Census Bureau. 2010. Idaho Quick Facts. Retrieved from <http://quickfacts.census.gov/qfd/states/16000.html>.

Winefield, H., Black, A. and Chur-Hansen, A. 2008. Health effects of ownership of and attachment to companion animals in an older population. *International Journal of Behavioral Medicine* 15: 303–310.

Wisdom, J. P., Saedi, G. A. and Green, C. A. 2009. Another breed of "service" animals: STARS study findings about pet ownership and recovery from serious mental illness. *American Journal of Orthopsychiatry* 79: 430–436.

Zeifman, D. and Hazan, C. 2008. Pair bonds as attachments: Reevaluating the evidence. In *Handbook of Attachment: Theory, Research, and Clinical Applications.* 2nd edn, 436–455, ed. J. Cassidy and P. R. Shaver. New York: Guilford.

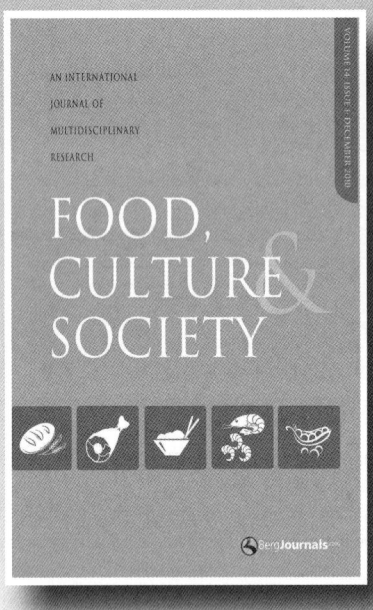
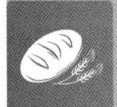 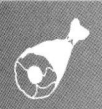   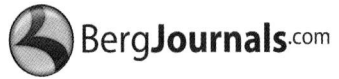

ANTHROZOÖS   VOLUME 25, ISSUE 1   REPRINTS AVAILABLE   PHOTOCOPYING   © ISAZ 2012
              PP. 121–124   DIRECTLY FROM   PERMITTED   PRINTED IN THE UK
                                   THE PUBLISHERS   BY LICENSING ONLY

NEWS AND ANALYSIS

New Books

The Psychology of the Human–Animal Bond: A Resource for Clinicians and Researchers

Edited by Chris Blazina, Güler Boyra and David Shen-Miller

This book offers a contextual framework for understanding the dynamics of human–animal relationships, both in the larger society and on the client level. An international panel of scholars and clinicians from across psychology (as well as from philosophy, literature, and other disciplines outside mental health) explores topics that will help professionals deepen their understanding of the human–animal relationship, translate this insight to practice, and consider questions of identity, attachment, and ethics. In topics ranging from the universal (health benefits of pet ownership) to the timely (the exploitation of fighting dogs), the reader gains perspective on the numerous factors that influence the bond between humans and animals, and the ways in which the bond reflects our own challenges as humans. Key areas of coverage include: Cultural and contextual issues; Psychological aspects of attachment and well-being; Bereavement, loss, and disenfranchised grief; Animal rights, abuse, and neglect; and Tests, measurements, current research issues, and future directions. This book will be of great interest and practical use to psychologists, clinical social workers, and rehabilitation professionals such as physical and occupational therapists. Published in 2011 by Springer. ISBN-13: 978-1441997609 (hardback).

Theorizing Animals: Re-thinking Humanimal Relations

Edited by Nik Taylor and Tania Signal

Utilizing ideas from post-modernism and post-humanism, this book challenges current ways of thinking about animals and their relationships with humans. Including contributions from across the social sciences, this book encourages readers to reflect upon taken-for-granted ways of conceptualizing human relationships with animals. It will be of interest to those in the broad field of human–animal studies, as well as those within most social science and humanities disciplines including sociology, anthropology, philosophy, and social theory. Published in 2011 by BRILL. ISBN-13: 9789004202429 (paperback).

Anthrozoös DOI: 10.2752/175303712X13240472427113

Loving Animals: Toward a New Animal Advocacy

By Kathy Rudy

Offering an alternative to both the acceptance of animal exploitation and radical animal liberation, Rudy shows that a deeper understanding of the nature of our feelings for and about animals can redefine the human–animal relationship in a positive way. Through extended interviews with people whose lives are intertwined with animals, analysis of the cultural representation of animals, and engaging personal accounts, she explores five realms in which humans use animals: as pets, for food, in entertainment, in scientific research, and for clothing. In each case she presents new methods of animal advocacy to reach a more balanced and sustainable relationship association built on reciprocity and connection. Published in 2011 by University of Minnesota Press. ISBN-13: 978-0-8166-7468-8 (hardback).

Living with Herds: Human–Animal Coexistence in Mongolia

By Natasha Fijn

Domestic animals have lived with humans for thousands of years and remain essential to the everyday lives of people throughout the world. In this book, Natasha Fijn examines the process of animal domestication in a study that blends biological and social anthropology, ethology, and ethnography. She examines the social behavior of humans and animals in a contemporary Mongolian herding society. After living with Mongolian herding families, Dr. Fijn has observed through firsthand experience both sides of the human–animal relationship. Examining their reciprocal social behavior and communication with one another, she demonstrates how herd animals influence Mongolian herders' lives and how the animals themselves are active partners in the domestication process. Published in 2011 by Cambridge University Press. ISBN-13: 9781107000902 (hardback).

Anthropocentrism: Humans, Animals, Environments

Edited by Rob Boddice

Anthropocentrism is a charge of human chauvinism and an acknowledgement of human ontological boundaries. Anthropocentrism has provided order and structure to humans' understanding of the world, while unavoidably expressing the limits of that understanding. This collection explores the assumptions behind the label "anthropocentrism," critically enquiring into the meaning of "human." It addresses the epistemological and ontological problems of charges of anthropocentrism, questioning whether all human views are inherently anthropocentric. In addition, it examines the potential scope for objective, empathetic, relational, or "other" views that trump anthropocentrism. With a principal focus on ethical questions concerning animals, the environment and the social, the essays ultimately cohere around the question of the non-human, be it animal, ecosystem, god, or machine. Published in 2011 by BRILL. ISBN-13: 9789004187948 (paperback).

Zoopolis: A Political Theory of Animal Rights

By Sue Donaldson and Will Kymlicka

Zoopolis offers a new agenda for the theory and practice of animal rights. Most animal rights theory focuses on the intrinsic capacities or interests of animals, and the moral status and moral rights that these intrinsic characteristics give rise to. *Zoopolis* shifts the debate from the realm of moral theory and applied ethics to the realm of political theory, focusing on the relational obligations that arise from the varied ways that animals relate to human societies and institutions. Building on recent developments in the political theory of group-differentiated citizenship, *Zoopolis* introduces us to the genuine "political animal." It argues that different types of animals stand in different relationships to human political communities. Published in 2011 by Oxford University Press. ISBN-13: 9780199599660 (hardback).

Conferences

British Animal Studies Network Meeting
Wild

May 25 to 26, 2012

This meeting will be held at the **University of Strathclyde, Glasgow, UK**. Some of the topics to be covered include: "The reintroduction of wild animals," "Wildness as a philosophical construct," and "Wild animals in captivity." Speakers include: Tim Ingold (University of Aberdeen), Hayden Lorimer (Glasgow University), and Richard Nash (Indiana University). For more information, go to the web site of the British Animal Studies Network: www.britishanimalstudiesnetwork.org.uk.

Animal Death

June 13, 2012

This symposium, to be held at the **University of Sydney, Australia**, brings together cross-disciplinary voices on the topic of Animal Death. The keynote speaker is Professor Deborah Bird Rose (Macquarie University, Australia). For further information, please contact the organizers: Dr Jay Johnston (jay.johnston@sydney.edu.au) and Dr Fiona Probyn-Rapsey (fiona.probyn-rapsey@sydney.edu.au).

UFAW Animal Welfare Conference
Recent Advances in Animal Welfare Science III

June 21, 2012

This conference of the Universities' Federation for Animal Welfare will be held in **York, UK** at the York Merchant Adventurers' Hall. It aims to provide a forum at which the broad community of scientists, veterinarians, and others concerned with animal welfare can come together to share knowledge and practice, discuss advances, and exchange views. Further details, including a registration form, can be found on the UFAW web site: www.ufaw.org.uk/conference2012.php.

9th Annual Symposium of the International Medieval Society-Paris

June 28 to 30, 2012

This symposium of the International Medieval Society in Paris (IMS-Paris) is organized around the theme of human/animal in medieval France. It will be held in **Paris, France** and will focus on a number of key questions:

- How was the relationship between human and animal conceptualized, represented and discussed in medieval cultural traditions (philosophical, literary, artistic, architectural, musical, or other)?

- What significance does the relationship and/or distinction between humans and animals have in the social and legal contexts in which they interacted?

- To what extent were human and animal thought of as separable or confusable categories? How is this related to behavioral, linguistic, physical, cultural, or other factors?

- In what ways does thinking about animals in the Middle Ages serve to define a notion of the human? Is it possible to conceive of the animal in a way that does not reflect on the human?

For more information, please go to: www.ims-paris.org.

Minding Animals 2012

July 4 to 6, 2012

This conference is the second in a series of conferences about scientific, ethical, and social issues related to human interactions with, and uses of, animals. It will be held at **Utrecht University, The Netherlands.** The aim of the conference is to bring together academics from different areas (animal welfare, animal ethics, and animal studies in general) and politicians and a broad variety of interest groups. The conference offers a platform for exchange of information about research developments, debates about controversial political and ethical issues concerning the treatment of animals, and a variety of cultural activities around animals. For further information, send an e-mail to: mindinganimals@uu.nl, or go to the web site: www.uu.nl/faculty/humanities/EN/congres/mindinganimals.

21st Annual ISAZ Conference
The Arts & Sciences of Human–Animal Interaction

July 11 to 13, 2012

This conference will be held at **Murray Edwards College, Cambridge, UK**. Topics which will be covered include:

- Animals and human–animal interaction in film, television, literature, music, and art

- Attitudes to animals and animal issues (contemporary and historical)

- The impact of human–animal interactions on the health and well-being of people and other animals

- Cultural studies of human–animal interaction

- Animal welfare and ethical issues

Early bird registration ends on **March 30, 2012**. More information can be found at: wwww.isaz2012.com, or send an e-mail to: conferences@isaz.net.

ANTHROZOÖS   VOLUME 25, ISSUE 1   REPRINTS AVAILABLE   PHOTOCOPYING   © ISAZ 2012
                     PP. 125–126   DIRECTLY FROM   PERMITTED   PRINTED IN THE UK
                                        THE PUBLISHERS   BY LICENSING ONLY

BOOK REVIEWS

Camel

Robert Irwin. London: Reaktion Books, 2010. 232 pages. ISBN: 978 1 86189 649 0 (paperback)

Reviewed by: Juliet Clutton-Brock, South Barn, High Street, Fen Ditton, Cambridge CB5 8ST, UK. E-mail: juliet.cb@btinternet.com
DOI:10.2752/175303712X13240472427078

 Camel follows the prescribed format of this burgeoning series of natural history books from Reaktion in having seven chapters and ending with detailed notes, a select bibliography, and a list of websites. Robert Irwin is a professional writer of distinction and an erudite scholar of Arabic literature, and as author of this book on camels it shows. The book runs smoothly through a huge number of fascinating anecdotes, quotations, and descriptions, nearly all of the one-humped camel or dromedary. Although Irwin is no biologist he has reviewed the scientific literature and the first chapter has a wealth of information about camel anatomy, physiology, and behavior, of both the dromedary and the Bactrian. The reader will learn about feeding, anatomy, mating behavior, loyalty to humans, and a great many other details, all of which are well illustrated, especially the two line drawings with names for parts of the body and skeleton. The chapter ends with the belief of a creationist that, "It is difficult to imagine how all the various features the camel needs in order to survive could have developed by gradual evolutionary processes." This is countered by Irwin's pertinent comment: "However, the argument from lack of imagination is not a strong one."

A short chapter follows on the fossil ancestors of the camel and its evolution in North and South America during the Pleistocene period. However, Irwin's explanation for the ecological distribution of the living species of camelids is surely unlikely: "The camel is a timid creature and is poorly equipped for defence from the predators. Its best defence has been to retreat to desert or mountainous areas … the dromedary and the Bactrian found their place in the desert. In South America, the camelids, comprising the llama, vicuna, alpaca and guanaco specialized in grazing at high altitudes."

The third chapter is called "Practical Camel" and rather surprisingly begins with advice on keeping a camel as a pet, and is then followed with instructions on how to ride a camel, on its normal speed of three miles an hour, on the different types of saddle, and on the gruesome act of inserting a nose peg, as camels cannot be ridden with a bit because they chew all the time. The chapter ends with slaughter and eating camel meat, with recipes for cooking. Although the camel chews the cud, it does not have a cloven hoof, so its meat is forbidden to Jews in the Old Testament Laws.

The camel's role in history would be expected to follow after its fossil history but this has had to wait until Chapter Six. It begins with the statement that there is no evidence for the history of the domestication of the camel. However, this is not true for there is now a considerable data-base of archaeozoological evidence for the where and when for domestication of the wild dromedary. For some years, Professor Hans-Peter Uerpmann and his wife Margarethe have been excavating the remains of one-humped camels from sites in South East Arabia and their reports and reviews are readily available on the Web. These authors conclude with considerable certainty that, in Arabia, the shift from hunting to herding camels occurred between about 1400 and 900 BCE.

The same authors suggest that the wild two-humped camel may have existed in the dry steppes and deserts of the Iranian Highland, where it may have been domesticated during the second millennium BCE, as possibly indicated by the early findings at the site of Shar-e-Sokhta. The chapters on the fossil history and early domestication of the camel may be weak, but the strength of this book lies not so much in the natural history of the camel but in its anthrozoology, that is the relationships and interactions between humans and camels, especially the dromedary. In the descriptions and images chosen to illustrate the place of these iconic beasts of burden in the history of Eastern and Western life, literature, and art, Robert Irwin excels, and fulfils the aim of the Reaktion animal series.

As Irwin states, from the second century BCE the Bactrian camel, as a pack animal, allowed the silk road from China to classical Rome to develop and achieve great importance for trade throughout the ancient world up to the first century CE. Camels were not used by the ancient Egyptians, but were present in Ptolemaic times (from 323 BCE) and are found on the rock art of North Africa from around 2,000 years ago. They are frequently mentioned in the Old Testament and in the Koran. The more recent history of the camel ranges over the Mamluk and Ottoman periods in the middle ages, to their use in Napolean's warfare, through their introduction to Australia in 1840, and their vital use by T. E. Lawrence in Arabia at the beginning of the twentieth century. It has been estimated that during the First World War 22,812 camels were killed on active service.

As an example of the Western, romantic image of Arabia and the camel, Irwin quotes my favorite opening lines to a novel, those of Rose Macauley's *The Towers of Trebizond* (1956), which perfectly sums up the fictional magic of the desert traveler: "'Take my camel dear,' said my aunt Dot, as she climbed down from the animal on her return from high mass. The camel, a white Arabian Dhalur (single hump) from the famous herd of the Ruola tribe, had been a parting present, its saddle bags stuffed with low-carat gold and flashy orient gems, from a rich desert tycoon."

Many descriptions and facts about the modern camel are given in the final chapter, and these include the wild Bactrian camel, which still exists in small numbers in the Gobi Desert, in the Lop Nor Wild Camel National Nature Reserve, and in captive breeding programs in China. Camel racing in the Arabian peninsula is viewed as a traditional sport but in fact it was inaugurated by King Fahd of Saudi Arabia in 1975, with today, prized dromedaries being exercised on treadmills and in swimming pools, and fed cow's milk and honey. Camel fighting and wrestling is an older sport and is illustrated with an eighteenth-century Mughal painting. Today, one-humped camels are common beasts of burden in India, and in East Africa they are bred for milk and meat, with large herds being owned by the nomadic pastoralists. Perhaps unexpectedly, in north-east Kenya the nomads have a Mobile Library Service with the camels carrying about 400 books.

Although, like all the Reaktion series, *Camel* is small in size, it has a large number of excellent illustrations and it is so well written and so full of fascinating facts and anecdotes that it will be particularly satisfying to read and own.

NOTES FOR CONTRIBUTORS

The following details should be used **as a guide only**. Full details can be found at the Berg Publishers web site: www.bergpublishers.com.

Content

Anthrozoös will accept new contributions that describe the characteristics and consequences of interactions/relationships between people and non-human animals. Papers are welcome from the arts and humanities, behavioral and biological sciences, social sciences, and the health sciences.

Types of Articles

Commentaries

This section provides a forum for raising issues related to the fields of interest of the Journal, including theory, methodology, ethics, statistical analysis, and nomenclature. Authors may make general points or provide critiques of particular published papers. These articles should usually be no longer than 5000 words.

Review Articles and Research Reports

Reviews—These should address fundamental issues related to the interactions between people and other animals, and provide new insights into the subject(s) they cover. Original interdisciplinary syntheses are especially welcome. Reviews should be no longer than 8000 words.

Research Reports—both quantitative and qualitative reports are encouraged. These should cover subjects falling within the scope of the Journal and can be up to 6000 words in length.

Note: Word counts do not include tables, figures and references.

Manuscript Submission

Only electronic submission of manuscripts is possible (please do not send by post). To submit a manuscript, go to: http://anthrozoos.expressacademic.org/login.php Electronic manuscripts must be in MS-Word (.doc files only—do not send .docx files) and sent as one file only (all text, tables, figures, and appendices in one file). Manuscripts **must not contain authors' names and addresses, and any acknowledgements section must be left blank.** Papers which are not formatted correctly may be returned to the author unread.

Authors whose first language is not English must have their paper checked by a native English speaker before submitting it.

Manuscript Organization

Use double-line spacing and align the text to the left. Use active voice whenever feasible and write in the first person. **American spelling and grammar conventions** must be used throughout, except in non-American quotations and references. Manuscripts should have line numbers and page numbers throughout.

The title page should contain the title of the article. In the following pages, provide an abstract (250 to 300 words), 3 to 5 keywords (in alphabetical order below the abstract), and the text, including, as appropriate, an introduction, methods, results, discussion, acknowledgements, notes, references, appendices, tables, figure captions, and figures. Each table/ figure must appear on a separate page.

Footnotes

Footnotes appear as "Notes" at the end of articles. Authors are advised to include footnote material in the text whenever possible. Notes are to be numbered consecutively throughout the paper and are to be typed, double-spaced at the end of the text (**do not** use any footnoting or end-noting programs that your text software may offer, as this text becomes irretrievably lost at the typesetting stage).

References

For references in the text, give full surnames for papers by one, two or three authors, but only the surname of the first author, followed by "et al." for four or more (note that "et al." is neither underlined nor italicized). Check that all references in the text are in the reference list and vice versa, and that their dates and spelling match. Check foreign language references particularly carefully for accuracy of diacritical marks such as accents and umlauts.

Cite references in the text as, for example, Swabe (1998) or, if in parentheses, as (Daly and Morton 2006) or (McGreevy, Righetti and Thomson 2005). **Do not** use a comma to separate the author's name from the date. Where more than one paper by the same author has appeared in one year, the reference should be distinguished by "a," "b," "c," etc. (e.g., 1971a). If referring to a specific page in a book, please provide the page number in the citation: for example, (Serpell 1999, p. 45). Where multiple citations are referred to, place in chronological order, from oldest paper to most recent, using a semicolon to separate each reference: for example, (Harrison 1998; Gibbs 1999; Bekoff 2006).

The list of references should be arranged alphabetically by authors' names and chronologically per author. References cited with "et al." in the text should include all authors' names in the reference list. Journal titles should be given in full. References to books or monographs should include editors, edition and volume number, publisher, city and state or country where published, and relevant page numbers. A paper in press may be referenced if it has been accepted for publication. References to personal communications and unpublished work should appear in the text only.

Sample references (note: do not indent):

Galvin, S. and Herzog, H. 1992. Ethical ideology, animal activism and attitudes towards the treatment of animals. *Ethics and Behavior* 2: 141–149.

Lennon, R. and Eisenberg, N. 1987. Gender and age differences in empathy and sympathy. In *Empathy and its Development*, 195–217, ed. N. Eisenberg and J. Strayer. New York: Cambridge University Press.

Philo, C. and Wilbert, C. eds. 2000. *Animal Spaces, Beastly Places: New Geographies of Human–Animal Relations*. London: Routledge.

Paul, E. S. 1992. Pets in childhood: individual variation in childhood pet ownership. Ph.D. thesis, University of Cambridge, UK.

Tables

Each table must be presented on a separate page and be identified by a short, descriptive title placed at the top. Any necessary further explanations (e.g., the results of statistical tests) may be added as footnotes at the base of the table. Make sure that each abbreviation used in a table is fully explained in a footnote. Marginal notations on manuscripts should indicate approximately where tables are to appear. Please use Helvetica or Arial font for all tables. Each table must be cited in the text.

Authors using MS-Word or other word-processing programs must use those programs' table editors to create tables. **Do not** create tables by typing single lines of text followed by a hard return, with spaces or tabs used to align columns.

Figures

All illustrative material (drawings, maps, diagrams, graphs and photographs) should be designated "Figures" and must be cited in the text. For the review process, it is acceptable to supply low-resolution figures. Once a paper is accepted, the author will be required to supply high-resolution files/prints of figures (electronic files are preferred). Figures will be reproduced exactly as provided. However, as they will be reduced in size to fit the Journal's page format, they must be of a size which will allow a reduction of 50%.

Track Changes

Some word-processing programs offer authors the ability to check the changes they have made to their manuscript after making revisions. In MS-Word, this is called "Track Changes." If you do use this or a similar utility, please remember to click "**accept all changes**" and deselect "**Track Changes**" before you submit your manuscript.

Criteria for Evaluation

Anthrozoös is refereed and papers will be accepted only after appropriate blind review. The general criteria for acceptance are that the research meet standards for publication in a specialty journal appropriate to its field and that it provide new information, sound hypotheses, or insightful analyses relevant to the content area of Anthrozoös. This is a multidisciplinary journal, and authors should be aware that their own discipline's jargon may be unfamiliar to readers from other disciplines. Please keep jargon to a minimum and provide a complete methods section. If you are in doubt about this, please err on the side of providing fuller explanations. The Editor can always cut material but cannot add it.

Ethical Considerations

Studies Involving Animals

If studies have the potential to compromise animal welfare, precautions should be taken to reduce possible harm to the animals involved. Authors should identify welfare concerns and describe the measures that were taken to mitigate animal pain or distress. *Anthrozoös* will not accept any manuscripts based on research inflicting suffering or cruelty on animals.

Studies Involving Humans

Informed consent should be given by persons participating in the studies reported. Any sensitive data should be handled with confidentiality and stored securely. When reporting results, participants should remain anonymous.

Conflicts of Interest

Any personal, financial, or other potential or actual conflicts of interest relating to the study should be conveyed by the authors.

Copyright

Papers are accepted on the understanding that they are subject to editorial revision and that they are contributed only to this Journal. Copyright in the article, including the right to reproduce the article in all forms and media, shall be assigned exclusively to the Journal. The transfer of copyright to Anthrozoös takes effect when the manuscript is accepted for publication.

Proofs

One set of proofs will be sent to the corresponding author as an e-mail attachment (PDF). Only typographic errors may be corrected at this stage.

On publication, authors will be sent a PDF e-print (with nonprinting watermark) of the final, published version of their article for personal use, and will be able to order a free copy of the issue in which their article appears through Berg Publishers. Contact Ken Bruce at ken.bruce@bloomsbury.com.

Contact

If you have any questions, please contact the Editor-in-Chief, Dr Anthony L. Podberscek: alp18@cam.ac.uk.